SAFEGUARDING CHILDREN & YOUNG PEOPLE

Sara Miller McCune founded SAGE Publishing in 1965 to support the dissemination of usable knowledge and educate a global community. SAGE publishes more than 1000 journals and over 800 new books each year, spanning a wide range of subject areas. Our growing selection of library products includes archives, data, case studies and video. SAGE remains majority owned by our founder and after her lifetime will become owned by a charitable trust that secures the company's continued independence.

Los Angeles | London | New Delhi | Singapore | Washington DC | Melbourne

SAFEGUARDING CHILDREN & YOUNG PEOPLE

A GUIDE FOR PROFESSIONALS WORKING TOGETHER

NICK FROST

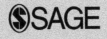

Los Angeles | London | New Delhi
Singapore | Washington DC | Melbourne

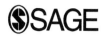

Los Angeles | London | New Delhi
Singapore | Washington DC | Melbourne

SAGE Publications Ltd
1 Oliver's Yard
55 City Road
London EC1Y 1SP

SAGE Publications Inc.
2455 Teller Road
Thousand Oaks, California 91320

SAGE Publications India Pvt Ltd
B 1/I 1 Mohan Cooperative Industrial Area
Mathura Road
New Delhi 110 044

SAGE Publications Asia-Pacific Pte Ltd
3 Church Street
#10-04 Samsung Hub
Singapore 049483

Editor: Kate Keers
Assistant editor: Ruth Lilly
Production editor: Martin Fox
Copyeditor: Jo North
Proofreader: Elaine Leek
Marketing manager: Camille Richmond
Cover design: Wendy Scott
Typeset by: C&M Digitals (P) Ltd, Chennai, India

Library of Congress Control Number: 2020937759

British Library Cataloguing in Publication data

A catalogue record for this book is available from
the British Library

ISBN 978-1-5264-9438-2
ISBN 978-1-5264-9437-5 (pbk)

CONTENTS

LIST OF FIGURES AND TABLES

Figures

Tables

ABOUT THE AUTHOR

Nick Frost is Emeritus Professor at Leeds Beckett University, UK. He was a local authority social worker and an adult educator, before joining Leeds Beckett University in 2009. Nick has over a decade of experience as Chair of three different Local Safeguarding Children Boards. He has addressed conferences on child welfare issues in many countries and acted as a consultant to a number of governments and voluntary organisations. Nick has produced over 20 books including *Understanding Children's Social Care* (with Nigel Parton, Sage, 2009) and *The Routledge Handbook of Global Child Welfare* (with Pat Dolan, Routledge, 2017).

ACKNOWLEDGEMENTS

I have valued the help provided by many people during the writing of this book. Thanks are due to:

Professor Nigel Parton for the initial idea and for being a supportive sounding board.

Dr Peter Mills who helped with the work on Jimmy Savile. Dr Tracey Race for her work on children, young people and parents' engagement with the child protection system, which I have drawn on extensively. Allison Waddell for useful, meticulous and very helpful comments on the text. Anonymous reviewers for all their constructive suggestions. All the staff and members of the three safeguarding boards that I have known well, and whose practice is both inspirational and innovative. The great staff team at Sage who have been helpful and informative throughout. And, last but not least, Dawn for being supportive of the project throughout.

INTRODUCTION

This book is aimed at the entire range of practitioners who work in the field of safeguarding children and young people, or students who are preparing to do so. These potentially include those working in health, social care, education, the police and the voluntary sector. The book is written from my experience and from the recognition that this work is both complex and demanding: the analysis sits quite squarely on the side of practitioners who undertake this very difficult and complex task. The book draws on the author's experience as a social worker, a researcher, a lecturer and, most significantly, over a decade of experience as the Chair of three different Local Safeguarding Children Boards (LSCBs). It is hoped that the book is equally relevant to all those who buy in to the phrase that 'safeguarding is everyone's business' and whose role is thus covered, in England, by the official guidance *Working Together to Safeguard Children* (HMG, 2018).

There are three key underlying arguments made in this book. One is that our understanding of child abuse is 'socially constructed' – that is, that it varies across time and space and the social response to child abuse varies considerably in different societal and political contexts. Second, it is proposed that professional practice can only be fully understood in a wider social, political and policy context. A focus on this context alone is sometimes unhelpful in guiding professional practice: and to focus on skills and knowledge, without the wider context, is in danger of failing to recognise the complex and challenging social environment in which practitioners deploy their skills. We need to place practice in the wider social context. The final key argument is that child protection practice often is situated on the border between the State (the public arena) and the household (the private arena) – this boundary between public and private is always difficult to negotiate in liberal democratic states and is a key reason why child protection is always complex, sometimes controversial, and often makes the news headlines. We have also learnt that abuse and maltreatment occur within localities and across national boundaries, presenting yet more complex challenges for practitioners.

The book aims to introduce the main elements of safeguarding children and young people – and provides a guide for further reading at the end of each chapter for readers if you require more breadth and depth on a specific topic. The book is structured as follows:

Chapter 1 provides 'a brief history of child protection'. The aim is to present a historical and social context, so we can focus on how the understanding of child abuse – and the resultant safeguarding system – has changed over time. When we work in a contemporary structure it is easy to imagine that the system is a given, something that is 'set in stone': but of course, it is not. Systems, knowledge, and understanding alongside political and social priorities alter over time and sometimes this change occurs rapidly. The chapter explores the roots of the current system, which are to be found in the Victorian era, and then analyses how this has developed into contemporary forms of organising and working in the child protection field.

Chapter 2 explores 'working together' to safeguard children, which deliberately draws on the title of the English government statutory guidance on child protection (HMG, 2018). We will explore a particular theory of multi-disciplinary working – that is, the theory proposed by the social learning theorist Etienne Wenger: it is suggested that this theory provides a useful framework for understanding how safeguarding can be truly multi-disciplinary, through the building of what Wenger defines as 'communities of practice'. The chapter also provides a critical commentary on the current strategic organisation of the leadership of safeguarding systems in England, systems which underpin direct practice.

Chapter 3 attempts to bring together theoretical understandings of child abuse and child protection. The chapter extends one of the key arguments of the book around the social construction of child abuse and the impact of these contested understandings on actual safeguarding practice. The chapter draws on international sources in order to work towards a global perspective (Dolan and Frost, 2017). A number of different theoretical positions are presented and critically analysed.

In Chapter 4 two case studies are provided to illustrate perceptions relating to differing forms of abuse: first there is a case study of 'celebrity abuse' based on the notorious British case of the disc jockey Jimmy Savile. The aim is not so much to dwell on the detail of Savile's crimes – but rather to understand the dynamics and the abuse of power which is still going on today. Second, there is a further case study of the abuse of children and young people in different institutional settings. Again there are particular dynamics which share features whether the abuse took place in large children's homes of the past or in contemporary sports teams or public schools. Both case studies are presented in depth as, it is argued, the debates and theories are transferable to other contexts where abuse takes place. It is necessary to present some quite upsetting detail in this chapter which the reader should hold in mind before reading these case studies.

Chapter 5 explores the crucial area of assessment and the provision of family support, referred to as 'early help' in the official English documentation. A value position of this book is that family support should always be central to safeguarding practice: and that the existence of a firewall between family support and safeguarding is both dangerous and damaging. The chapter argues for an assessment process which is pro-active and inclusive, drawing on the establishment of positive, relationship-based practice.

Chapter 6 outlines the nature of safeguarding practice on the front-line. Drawing on the more theoretical work earlier in this book the chapter explores safeguarding practice – exploring the crucial role of the home visit, relationship-based practice and multi-disciplinary working. The chapter is more applied than the previous chapters, exploring both prevention and intervention, whilst analysing some useful approaches to working with children, young people and their families.

Chapter 7 explores the most recent high-profile issue in safeguarding which began with a focus on child sexual exploitation and which has developed, more recently, into what has been identified as a contextual approach to safeguarding. The chapter explores theories, policy directions and the practice implications in relation to child sexual exploitation.

Chapter 8 moves on to analyse contextual safeguarding, a contemporary development in the safeguarding field. This is a crucial shift in a focus from the family context of abuse in order to take into account the wider community context. The emergent implications for policy and practice are explored here.

Chapter 9 brings together, in a hopefully practical manner, the skill set required by front-line practitioners: the home visit and the role of reflection and supervision, for example. This chapter also covers some issues that are often not discussed by safeguarding texts – including the conduct and chairing of safeguarding meetings.

The book concludes by bringing together the main themes, reflecting on our key arguments and critically assessing the current 'state of the art' in terms of safeguarding children and young people.

There are some technical issues of expression and explanation that should be noted at this stage. First, it is legally correct to refer to all people under 18 as 'children'. In this text we use children and young people when the discussion refers to all under 18s: we use the term 'children' when we are referring to the younger age range and 'young people' when we discuss the older age range of young people. The term adolescent is not used as this tends to have a pejorative meaning attached to it. Second, the author's experience is mainly based in England: but within the United Kingdom there is now a complex devolution of powers to Northern Ireland, Scotland and Wales. It would be very demanding to constantly list these differences in policy and practice. International sources are used throughout and where the English policy is outlined the international reader should be able to transfer the analysis to whichever national context they are working in.

The book tries to achieve two overall intentions: first, to provide a direction of good safeguarding practice, whilst simultaneously arguing that such practice cannot exist only in a technical, procedural sense as safeguarding needs to be informed by social theory, social history and political analysis. It is argued that the practitioner never exists in isolation but in a series of interactions with a complex and changing social environment. One implication of this is that professional learning is a lifelong process of information gathering and critical reflection.

Second, safeguarding is perceived in both the wider and the narrower sense. In the wider sense we explore the fundamental policy shifts that are required if children and young people are to have better lives: exploring issues such as poverty, gender inequality, discrimination related to disability, generation and sexuality. We also look at safeguarding in the more focused sense: the dilemmas facing practitioners world-wide when they are concerned about a specific child on, say, a Monday morning. It is hoped that the book makes a meaningful contribution towards addressing the challenge of effectively safeguarding children and young people.

1

A BRIEF HISTORY OF CHILD PROTECTION

CONTENTS

This chapter aims to:

- Argue that child abuse and child protection practices are socially constructed
- Explore the tensions between 'care' and 'control'
- Propose that our understanding of contemporary practices can be improved by an understanding of social history
- Explore the roots of current child protection forms of practice

Introduction

One of the key premises of this book is that our understanding of, and response to, child abuse is 'socially constructed': that is that these understandings and practices change across time and place in a complex relationship with the wider social and political context. This is not simply a theoretical or academic point – understanding social construction has a direct impact on our practice. For example, although causation is complex, it is undoubtedly the case that the number of children subject to care proceedings and subsequently in the care system in England, increased after the publicity following the death of 'Baby Peter' (Jones, 2014). Arguably then, there is somewhere a mechanism whereby practitioners, their managers and, subsequently, CAFCASS (the Children and Family Court Advisory and Support Service) and the family courts respond differently to safeguarding situations after a high level of media coverage than prior to this coverage. This provides an example of how professional responses to child protection are subject to forms of active 'social construction'. This chapter takes a wider historical lens to examine these important processes of social change further.

Understanding the history of childhood

We cannot understand the history of child abuse without exploring the history of childhood more generally: childhood, parenting and child abuse form a complex and ever-changing Venn diagram (Wright, 2015). A long historical perspective is taken by the psycho-historian of childhood Lloyd DeMause, who argues that:

> Infanticide during antiquity has usually been played down despite literally hundreds of clear references by ancient writers that it was an accepted, everyday occurrence. (1974: 25)

There can be no doubt, as DeMause argues, that child abuse has existed since the beginning of humankind: there will have been acts of neglect and cruelty towards children and young people committed in many early civilisations. For example, in a society known for its sophistication and philosophy – Ancient Greece – there is historical documentation that illustrates older males had anal sex with younger boys, whom we would now describe as 'under age'. This was known at the time, was in the public arena and was well documented (Ungaretti, 1978). Today we would name these very same acts as 'child sexual exploitation' or 'grooming'. Another example comes from the slave trade. The slave trade is often written about and portrayed in dramas and films, but is rarely seen through the lens of child abuse. There is clear evidence that children were exploited for their labour and that this included physical abuse, but there is also evidence that young women were also sexually exploited and raped by slave owners and their employees (see Warren, 2007, for example). Again, today we would argue that these children and young people were subject to organised sexual exploitation.

From these sources – and there are numerous others – it can be argued that children and young people have been significantly exploited throughout history: what has varied is the nature of this abuse as well as the social, political and legal responses to it. We move on to explore how child protection as a modern social practice changed and developed in the period from 1850 onwards.

Creating modern safeguarding practice: the Victorian era

It is in the Victorian era, in Great Britain and the United States, that (during the latter half of the nineteenth century) we can find the roots of contemporary child protection practice. During this period, we can perceive the emergence of a range of foundational child welfare practices including the home visit, the case record and the early formulations of multi-agency working, and the resultant focus on abuse within the household.

There is a considerable historical debate about childhood and when it was 'discovered'. To say childhood was 'discovered' at first seems counter-intuitive: surely babies and children have existed throughout the history of humanity? Of course, biological children have always existed but 'childhood' is a social concept, referring to a protected social space, where younger people grow, develop and are educated. The social historian Philippe Ariès (1965) argued that the first evidence of childhood in this sense emerged during the seventeenth century – he uses sources such as diaries, paintings and official records to suggest that childhood became a space for play, nurturing and education, often, but not always, accompanied by parental care and affection. This proposal that children were often maltreated is controversial amongst social historians and is disputed by many, including the eminent historical scholar Linda Pollock (1983). Pollock argues, using diaries as a major source of evidence, that parental affection has a longer, consistent (and perhaps biologically based) history.

Whatever the outcome of this intense historical debate there is no doubt that by the 1840s childhood existed as an identifiable social space, certainly amongst the upper and middle class – a gendered experience that included play, education and elements of protection (Cunningham, 2014; Wright, 2015). The space for children of the toiling classes, in agriculture or emerging industry, was different: it was often risky, harsh and very hard work. At the start of the nineteenth century, during the 1800s, there was little welfare provision for children. The Thomas Coram Foundling Hospital was formed in London in 1739 and was perhaps the first child welfare institution as such: originally designed to house abandoned babies it soon developed a wider function of raising children whose mothers could not care for them (Pugh, 2011). The Coram Hospital is exceptional and more usually child welfare was an undifferentiated part of adult provision administered through the Poor Law.

Later in the nineteenth century a comprehensive welfare system was in place – codified in the 1889 Children Act, which is sometimes known as 'the Children's Charter'. In 1908 incest was made illegal by the Punishment of Incest Act and a more comprehensive Children Act was passed during the same year (Stewart, 1995). Thus, we can ask what happened between 1850 and 1908 to bring about these fundamental changes in attitudes, law and practice in relation to child-hood, child welfare and child abuse, which in turn led to the emergence of a child welfare system?

The emergence of a child protection system

As childhood emerged as an identifiable social space concern grew, particularly amongst the newly emergent middle classes, that the protections of middle-class childhood were not available for all children. In the rapidly growing cities the middle classes witnessed children who lived on the streets and children being subject to inadequate parenting. The middle classes perceived child abuse to be a result of parental alcohol abuse, 'immorality' and 'fecklessness'. These concerns were expressed in newspaper columns and at meetings in both Great Britain and the United States of America. In New York, the roots of the Societies for the Prevention of Cruelty to Children (SPCCs) can be found. According to some social historians (although the facts are disputed, see Watkins, 1990) in 1873 a little girl called Mary Ellen was known to be neglected and severely abused by her father. Some concerned citizens tried to protect her but found they could only do so under the then animal protection laws. This incident contributed to the formation of the New York SPCC, in 1875, a model that was then exported to England, following a visit by a banker, T.F. Agnew, which led to Liverpool founding its own SPCC in 1883 (Allen and Morton, 1961).

Underlying the growth of the SPCCs, and other philanthropic organisations, there was a genuine (often Evangelical) motive alongside a concern about preventing social disorder (Stedman Jones, 2014) that led to these developments. The US historian Linda Gordon is particularly useful in helping us reflect on these issues. In her brilliant and highly recommended study *Heroes of Their Own Lives* (1988) Gordon utilises original case files from the SPCC workers, in and around Boston, Massachusetts, to explore how families were worked with from the 1880s until the 1950s: her research provides valuable insights into the values and approaches adopted by this early form of child protection work. Linda Gordon argues that the SPCCs developed partially as:

> helping children assumed a special resonance ... because children were thought to be innocent ... protecting children from the wrongs of adults unified the charitable and the controlling aspects. (1988: 29)

By 1885 the British National Society for the Prevention of Cruelty to Children (NSPCC) was formed and soon covered much of England. The aims of the NSPCC at this stage were as follows:

a   To prevent the public and private wrongs of children and the corruption of their morals

b   To take action for the enforcement of laws for their protection.

> (Allen and Morton, 1961: 112)

The NSPCC utilised paid staff, but also volunteers, to visit families where concerns had been expressed, often by neighbours and sometimes by the family members themselves. The NSPCC operated through street work, monitoring and home visits to ensure the welfare and protection of children. These early child protection officers were often ex-armed forces males who travelled on horseback across extensive areas to visit and monitor households:

> A tradition has grown up over the years for men who have retired from the Armed Services ... to form a large proportion of the Inspectorate, their knowledge of their fellow men and their power being valuable qualities of their work. (Allen and Morton, 1961: 136)

Females were originally volunteers, known as Women Visitors, who assisted the male Inspectors. The written reports of the early SPCC workers reveal an authoritarian approach, backed by moral judgements and a strong determination to protect children. Gordon's work shows that the early American SPCC records 'called clients

shiftless, coarse, low type, uncouth, immoral, feeble-mined, lazy and worthless'
(Gordon, 1988: 15). This demonstrates a social gap between workers and clients, as
well as a clearly judgemental approach. It raises issues about forms of 'care' and
'control' and leads us to ask to what degree safeguarding practitioners are caring for
people or are they attempting to control behaviour?

Related to this point about care and control are contemporary issues arising from
our discussion of social history – that is, how safeguarding officers dealt with social
differences, such as class, disability, gender and ethnicity. Gordon argues that the
SPCC workers were often confronting maltreatment of women and children by
men: men who often abused alcohol. The SPCCs undertook this task by 'society
workers ... [spending] most of their time on the streets and calling upon families in
their homes' (Gordon, 1988: 48). As we have already discussed, the Inspectors in
this early period of the SPCCs 'were almost always male, while the clients were
virtually all female' (Gordon, 1988: 14). Gordon further argues – contrary to the
argument of those who see social work as a form of social control (see Garrett, 2010,
for example) – that the workers tried to transfer power within the household
towards women and children: she emphasises 'the active role of agency' (1988: 296)
of the women and children, a theme we elaborate upon in Chapter 8. Gordon outlines family scenarios that (apart from the period detail) would be familiar to any
contemporary front-line worker:

> Windows dirty, curtains dirty, floor and everything else in the room dirty ...
> a fountain syringe was hanging on the wall and a vessel which was in an
> unsanitary condition was sitting on the floor. (Gordon, 1988: 88)

Interestingly, given some of the debates underpinning this book, we can describe their
primary approach as being based in 'family support', by which we mean the preference was for children to remain at home with their parents as opposed to some form
of alternative care. Unlike other charities established around the same time (National
Children's Homes and Dr Barnardo's) the NSPCC did not build extensive institutions
for the care of children. For a short period (1891–1903) they did have some
'children's shelters' and the NSPCC did, indeed, take parents to court – but by
preference they used what one prominent supporter called 'kindly remonstrance'
and argued that 'prevention is better than punishment' (Hesba Stretton, quoted in
Frost and Stein, 1989: 45) to try to reform errant parents. The issue of 'family support',
as against 'child protection', can be seen to underpin the history of child welfare,
and will be referred to throughout this book.

What is of particular interest to us in this context is how Linda Gordon reflects on
the interface between the SPCC staff and the families they worked with in terms of
social class and ethnicity. The context for the early part of the study is the USA of the

nineteenth century, which was an emerging industrial society based on the labour of migrant families drawn from across Europe and former slaves. In this context Gordon argues that the SPCC embodied White Anglo-Saxon Protestant (WASP) values: values that included hard work, cleanliness, sexual morality and sobriety. Using her meticulous study of the case records Gordon argues that the SPCC staff worked hard to get client families to aspire to these WASP values: the Inspectors assessed the cleanliness of houses, encouraged a household model where the male was the breadwinner and the woman the home maker, and discouraged domestic violence and alcohol consumption. This was a WASP model – but one which also empowered and protected women and children. Gordon's arguments are highly relevant to modern debates about anti-discriminatory practice and equalities in safeguarding practice.

In England Harry Ferguson has used a similar methodology to that adopted by Linda Gordon to explore child abuse and protection. His theorisation is consistent with that of Gordon but Ferguson develops a stronger focus on child protection work as a form of modern social change, expressed through the growth of bureaucratic forms of organisation and mobility. He also notes the interface with childhood distress as follows:

> as soon as they hit the streets, SPCC workers ... confronted the immediacy of how not only sight, but every other sense was brought to bear on practice, especially smell and touch and then really how vulnerable children and families actually lived ... and died. (Ferguson, 2004: 30)

Gordon's work, and the comparable work of Ferguson in Great Britain, demonstrates how child protection work is political – by which we mean that it always contains within it the exercise of power and the deployment of dominant social values. These profound historical and theoretical insights will inform the remainder of this book.

Reflection point

We have seen that in their work Gordon and Ferguson utilise their studies of original case records from the late nineteenth century (1880–1900) to argue that child protection work carries within it explicit dominant social values which both underpin and inform practice.

Thinking about a geographical area that you know:

1   What are the prevailing social values in that area?
2   Do the practitioners in that area reflect that local culture?
3   Do practitioners challenge elements of the local culture?

What are the implications of the dominant social values for your safeguarding practice?

Post-Second World War developments

The phrase that child protection is 'socially constructed' can be illustrated further by a discussion of developments in child protection since the end of the Second World War (1939–45). We have seen that the Victorian philanthropists and SPCCs raised the profile of child protection issues between the 1860s and the passage of the 1908 Children Act, in Great Britain. Arguably between the two World Wars (1918 until 1939) these child protection issues had a lower public and political profile:

> there remains to be explained the curious decline in public interest in child abuse between 1914 and the early 1960s. (Behlmer, 1982: 225)

Linda Gordon (1988) argues that this decline in interest was connected with an increased focus on economic well-being and concern about the plight of male bread-winners during the inter-war/Depression period. This level of focus and interest was to change partially due to the work led by C. Henry Kempe, at a hospital in Colorado, in the USA.

Kempe was a paediatrician who viewed X-rays of children who had suffered fractures. Kempe found that some of the children had experienced past fractures, which had not been reported and had self-healed (Parton, 2017). This led Kempe to make further inquiries where he concluded that some of the children had been subject to physical abuse (Lynch, 1985). Krugman and Korbin, in their appreciation of Kempe's work, identify the concept of 'battered baby syndrome' as being both 'provocative' and 'anger provoking' (2012: 23). Kempe was met with disbelief, and some personal abuse, but went on to establish that parental physical abuse was a reality. Kempe founded a research centre and, following the earlier SPCC model of the 1860s, his work was then developed in Great Britain – led by the NSPCC. In 1968 the NSPCC opened Denver House, in recognition of the work of Kempe in Denver, Colorado: this in turn led to research and practice with a focus on the physical abuse of children from the late 1960s onwards. This development was initially research-led but was soon to be overtaken by policy and practice change responding largely to 'scandals' and child abuse inquiries (Parton, 1985).

There are many studies which outline the developments from 1970 until 2015 in detail (see Parton, 2010, for example): here we take a more thematic approach. There are three key themes which emerge during this period:

1   Scandal-led policy making
2   An increasing emphasis on multi-disciplinary working
3   More detailed and prescriptive policy making.

We develop each of these themes in turn in the discussion below.

1   Scandal-led policy making has already been mentioned in this book. It is noteworthy that policy making in child welfare can often be related to the names of individual children – in a way that happens only rarely in, for example, the field of adult social care. As we have seen we can locate the commencement of child protection practice in the story (or perhaps the myth) of Mary Ellen in New York in 1873. The modern era of this style of practice policy and change can then be traced through the deaths of many children, such as Denis O'Neill (report published 1945), Maria Colwell (report published 1974), Tyra Henry (report published 1987), Kimberley Carlile (report published 1987), Jasmine Beckford (report published 1985), Victoria Climbié (report published 2003) and 'Baby Peter' Connelly (report published 2009). These are some of the most high-profile deaths which gathered considerable media coverage and related political responses: policy changes often followed from these deaths (Parton, 2017). There are also official reports into more wide-ranging occurrences which can also be significant in relation to policy making – most noteworthy of these are the Butler-Sloss Report into alleged sexual abuse in the Middlesbrough area of England (then known as Cleveland), published in 1988, and which contributed significantly to the development of the Children Act 1989; and a comparable report produced by Professor Alexis Jay on child sexual exploitation (CSE) in Rotherham and published in 2014. The Jay Report in turn contributed to a step-change in British responses to CSE. These child death reviews and the more wide-ranging reports, led legal, policy and practice development from 1972 until 2010. The question to be asked here is whether scandal-led policy leads to effective law and policy reforms? The response to the scandal tends to be short-term and often follows the 'moral panic' model outlined by the sociologist Stan Cohen (1972) in relation to youth groups known as 'mods' and 'rockers'. Cohen outlines how an incident becomes headline news, this then leads to a high-profile political reaction and clarion calls for 'something to be done'. This rapid knee-jerk policy making is not always effective. Further, returning to child protection, it seems rather strange that law and policy is led by a single 'bad case' rather than the thousands of examples of good practice that could be utilised. The scandal-led model also contradicts the calls often made by politicians and others for 'evidence-based policy'.

2   One theme that emerges in all the aforementioned reports are problems with multi-disciplinary working (MDW), inter-agency planning and information sharing. One observation often made about inquiries into child deaths is that the same issues are often explored in a range of reports. Frequently mentioned is that there have been problems with coordination

between services and there has also been a lack of information sharing. Such a shortfall in effective multi-disciplinary working can be seen in many of the key reports including, for example, the Cleveland report which outlined a lack of cooperation between the police, medical staff and social workers (Butler-Sloss, 1988). A similar theme of poor information sharing can be seen in reports on individual deaths – the Serious Case Reviews (SCRs) relating to Tyra Henry, Victoria Climbié and Baby Peter being amongst the numerous examples that could be provided. These findings have led to an increased official focus on improving forms of multi-disciplinary working (Frost and Robinson, 2016). This issue is highlighted, of course, in the title of the of the various versions of the government guidance *Working Together to Safeguard Children*: in the current everyday parlance 'safeguarding is everyone's business'. A recurrent theme of *Working Together to Safeguard Children* is outlining how each organisation and profession has a distinct role in safeguarding children, but that these should be coordinated locally, at various historical periods, by Area Review Committees, Area Child Protection Committees, Local Safeguarding Children Boards and currently by the Multi-Agency Safeguarding Arrangements: these bodies that, quite literally, bring organisational leaders together in one room, in order to ensure that they are working together as efficiently and effectively as possible.

3   The issues mentioned above in (a) and (b) contributed to more extensive and more prescriptive guidance which culminated in the 2015 version of *Working Together to Safeguard Children* (HMG, 2015). The reading of the child death reports from Maria Colwell onwards was that strong and prescriptive guidance was required to ensure that child abuse deaths were minimised. As Nigel Parton (2010) has outlined, over the decades this guidance became both more prescriptive and increasingly lengthy – particularly in the early years of the twenty-first century. This prescriptive approach can be problematic: it has arguably made child protection over-bureaucratic and procedural rather than relationship-based in approach (see Featherstone et al., 2014 and 2018, for a critique of these procedurally led approaches). This was certainly the case during the New Labour period in the UK (1997–2010) when significant increases in policy initiatives and expenditure on children was accompanied by rigorous regimes of audit and inspection (Frost and Parton, 2009). The emphasis during this period on following procedure and keeping to prescribed timescales led to what can be described as 'robotic' forms of practice – overseen by the threat of a negative Ofsted report which resulted in the downfall of many senior staff across the nation.

━━━━━━━━━ **Reflection point** ━━━━━━━━━━━━━━━━━━━━━

During the period of your career, or your training, what have been the main forces that have developed child safeguarding policy and practice?

Do these map on to points (a)–(c) above, or are they different?

We can see then following the research-led emergence of physical abuse as the primary policy focus in the 1960s we then entered a period of what can be called scandal-led, or inquiry-led, policy and practice changes which dominated British child protection practice from 1972 until around 2015. The policy story from 2015 onwards is picked up in the next chapter.

Conclusion

This chapter has:

- Argued that child abuse and child protection practices are socially constructed
- Explored the tensions between 'care' and 'control'
- Proposed that our understanding of contemporary practices can be improved by an understanding of social history
- Explored the roots of current child protection forms of practice.

By drawing on important work, by social historians such as Gordon and Ferguson, we have gained insights into the origins of child protection practice. It has been argued that we can understand our current forms of practice using this historical perspective. We have also seen that controversies – for example, about ethnicity, social class and social control – have a long history that helps us to understand some of our current challenges. Since the 1950s, first physical child abuse, and later child sexual abuse and then child sexual exploitation dominated policy and practice agendas. The trends towards scandal-led policy making, increased emphasis on multi-disciplinary working and increased proceduralism continued and examining these trends helps us to understand the current state of child protection policy and practice.

Recommended reading

Nigel Parton, *The Politics of Child Abuse* (1985)

Parton brilliantly outlines the political and social response to the death of Maria Colwell, an early example of a child death report that led to key policy and practice reforms. Parton's model works in terms of understanding responses to child deaths and child death inquiries that have occurred since the death of Maria in 1973. A classic text and well worth reading.

Linda Gordon, *Heroes of Their Own Lives* (1988)

Gordon's book is a stimulating and original read that draws on case records maintained in the early years of the Massachusetts Society for the Prevention of Cruelty to Children. Gordon maps in detail the work of the early child protection practitioners and she argues that this form of safeguarding work cannot be seen simply as social control, as it worked to empower abused women and children. A surprisingly easy book to read, which also provides powerful insight into contemporary safeguarding practice.

Harry Ferguson, *Protecting Children in Time* (2004)

Using a similar methodology to Linda Gordon, Ferguson's study explores the early records of the English NSPCC. His book is more heavily theorised than that of Gordon, as he argues that child protection operates as part of modernity, and that it is closely linked to ideas of mobility and risk. Ferguson provides valuable insights which, as in the case of Gordon, can be applied to current practice.

2

'WORKING TOGETHER' TO SAFEGUARD CHILDREN AND YOUNG PEOPLE

CONTENTS

The aims of this chapter are to:

- Utilise the theoretical model of 'communities of practice' to reach a critical assessment of multi-disciplinary working
- Explore the current system of organising and planning the safeguarding system, utilising the English example
- Critically assess the current system for enhancing multi-disciplinary working

Introduction

This chapter will, first of all, provide a theoretical context for multi-disciplinary working – drawing on Etienne Wenger's 'communities of practice' concept, which it is argued is applicable to child safeguarding work. The second aim is to explore how practitioners actually work together – this will draw primarily on the official guidance for England, *Working Together to Safeguard Children* (HMG, 2018). The chapter draws on the author's decade of experience of chairing Local Safeguarding Children Boards (LSCBs) and will cover issues relating to leadership and systems change.

Building a 'community of practice'

It is argued here that the concept of 'communities of practice' (Wenger, 1999) works well in outlining what effective safeguarding should look like: this framework has been applied by the author of this book in a variety of organisational settings. Wenger (1999), in his original research, observed the operation of a medical claims team to assess how effective and efficient team working and cooperation comes about. He defines the communities of practice he observed as follows:

> Communities of practice are groups of people who share a concern or a passion for something they do and learn how to do it better as they interact regularly. (www.wenger-trayner.com, accessed 17 March 2020)

Wenger's work is extensive, and worthy of further study, but in summary three key concepts that are relevant here are as follows: joint enterprise, mutual engagement and shared repertoire (Wenger, 1999). We will explore the deployment of these concepts and how they can be applied to child safeguarding practice.

'Joint enterprise' is the first of these concepts which can be applied in the safeguarding field. By joint enterprise Wenger means that participants share an agreed goal and purpose – that is, they are working together towards a joint enterprise. In the private sector this may be relatively straightforward, i.e. to maximise profit, although there may also be subsidiary goals. In terms of this book the most apparent and obvious joint enterprise is to safeguard children and young people. Whilst this may seem straightforward this is actually complex to put into practice and may involve contested and contrasting multi-professional perspectives. Thus, a joint enterprise may contain within it some tensions and/or different routes to the shared agreed goal. According to Wenger the aim of having a joint enterprise should not be to do away with conflict. As long as conflict and differences of opinion are handled well then constructive differences can contribute to more effective and considered action. In Chapter 9 of this book we discuss how chairing and meeting skills can be deployed to address differences and to ensure that joint enterprise works well to safeguard children and young people, thus building a more effective community of practice.

Wenger's second key concept is that of 'mutual engagement'. This concept can also be applicable to safeguarding and implies that all relevant parties are fully committed to, and pro-actively engaged with, the safeguarding task. This is important at all three operational levels: governmental, local agency and case holder level. At governmental level, inter-departmental cooperation, for example, in England between the Department for Education and the Department of Health and Social Care, a commitment to 'joining-up' and the provision of adequate resources are required to demonstrate mutual engagement. At the local authority level all lead partners – the police, clinical commissioning group and the local authority – and all the 'relevant agencies' identified by *Working Together to Safeguard Children* (HMG, 2018) need to be 'mutually engaged' and committed to the safeguarding task. In playing the role of a Chair of LSCBs I found this concept useful in thinking about whether or not an agency was fully engaged in the safeguarding process and when they should be challenged about a potential lack of engagement. At the case level this same process applies: we can ask 'are all practitioners mutually engaged in the specific case being discussed and actions being shared?'

Wenger's third key concept is that of 'shared repertoire'. This concept is more difficult to pin down than the previous two concepts: a repertoire involves intangible elements such as culture, language, humour as well as more concrete manifestations such as shared procedures, thresholds and paperwork. The shared repertoire grows over time and develops through practitioners actually 'working together'. An example, in child protection work, may come from generating a shared assessment process which all relevant agencies find useful and relevant. The cultural level – such as the use of humour and the other informal aspects of multi-disciplinary working – is also crucial in building effective communities of practice. When we are novice practitioners, in the first few months of working, we are in a period of observing any new setting: gradually we will become part of this culture ourselves and will help to shape the working of a community of practice. Crucially, for Wenger, these communities of practice are environments where practitioners learn, reflect and develop their own professional practice.

Having explored the application of the 'communities of practice' concept it is strongly argued here that effective child protection work can be seen as resting on communities of practice that work well in safeguarding children and young people.

Reflection point

Think of a case, a team or an organisation you know well. Using Wenger's framework, we can ask how well are the team working together?

Is there a shared sense of purpose – a joint enterprise?

Do people work together – is mutual engagement demonstrated?

Is there a shared culture – a shared repertoire – in terms of working tools and organisational culture?

What actions could be taken to overcome any shortcomings that you have identified?

Working together to safeguard children and young people

Safeguarding children and young people is probably the area of social and health care practice where multi-disciplinary working is the most developed. This trend towards multi-disciplinary working has drawn, largely, on learning from child death reports – in the modern era dating back to the report on the death of Maria Colwell published in 1974. This learning has been embedded in the now many iterations of *Working Together to Safeguard Children*, with the contemporary version being published in 2018 (HMG, 2018).

The approach to multi-disciplinary working has many levels – at governmental level (mainly between the Department for Education, Home Office and Department of Health and Social Care), at senior leadership level in each local authority area and in relation to individual cases between front-line practitioners. It is often argued that multi-disciplinary working facilitates information sharing, policy and practice development and produces more effective safeguarding for children and young people: an argument that will be explored further here. This chapter now explores how current arrangements are configured and provides a critical commentary on contemporary state of play.

The background to the contemporary organisational context

In 2016 the English government asked Alan Wood, a former Director of Children's Services, to undertake a review of the role of Local Safeguarding Children Boards (LSCBs), the body which was then accountable for multi-disciplinary working in safeguarding children and young people for each local authority area. The terms of reference for Wood's task were as follows:

> to lead a fundamental review of the role and functions of Local Safeguarding Children Boards (LSCBs) within the context of local strategic multi-agency working. (Wood, 2016: 1)

The need for 'a fundamental review' seemed to rest in a political view that the English safeguarding system was in many ways 'failing', and the inevitable consequence of this can be seen in the wording of the terms of reference. The view about the failing system had been expressed by Michael Gove and Edward Timpson when they were, in turn, the senior and junior Ministers responsible for the child protection system (see Frost, 2016). The Ministers had concerns about the quality of some Serious Case Reviews (SCRs) and were also concerned about the gradings made of LSCBs following Ofsted inspections. One aim of this chapter is to challenge this argument: a positive case is made for a safeguarding system that, despite many challenges, was functioning to a high standard, as are most of the practitioners employed within the system. As well as this positive view challenging a dominant populist political agenda it also opposes the arguments of some left-leaning academics who argue that the current system is not working well (see Featherstone et al., 2014, 2018).

Alan Wood undertook his review over a nine-month period and in relation to the future of LSCBs he reached the following conclusion:

> Overall, the responses I have received make clear to me that the case for fundamental reform is based on a widely held view that LSCBs, for a variety of reasons, are not sufficiently effective. The limitations of LSCBs in delivering their key objectives have been fully exposed in this review and by the work of Ofsted. There needs to be a much higher degree of confidence that the strategic multi-agency arrangements we make to protect children are fit-for-purpose, consistently reliable and able to ensure children are being protected effectively. (Wood, 2016: 5–6)

The Wood Review was published in May 2016, simultaneously with the government response, which accepted all the Wood proposals for change in full. The government response to the Wood Review stated that it aimed to achieve the following for the child protection system:

- Excellent practice is the norm;
- Partner agencies hold one another to account effectively;
- There is early identification of 'new' safeguarding issues;
- Learning is promoted and embedded;
- Information is shared effectively;
- The public can feel confident that children are protected from harm. (DfE, 2016: 4)

This response is rather flawed not least because it is impossible for a 'norm' to be excellent, as excellence actually means being above the norm. It is remarkable that a team of civil servants would allow such an error to be published in an official report, but as Freud identified in his *Psychopathology of Everyday Life* (1901) errors often have hidden meanings – and the meaning here is that the goal set for a child protection system is indeed impossible (that is, for excellence to be the norm). Apart from this crass error the aims are largely uncontroversial, although the final bullet point about public confidence is less apparent in the final version of official guidance (see HMG, 2018). The methods chosen for working towards the objectives of the Wood Review raised some challenging leadership issues and initiated a major process of change, during the 2016–2019 period. This change process restructured the leadership and architecture of the child safeguarding system.

The Wood Review, the government response and *Working Together to Safeguard Children* (HMG, 2018) seem to adopt a narrow focus on 'learning' which appears to focus largely on learning from reports in relation to serious incidents, rather than the wider professional development argued for throughout this text. In relation to the previous system of Serious Case Reviews (SCRs) the government response to Wood argued as follows:

> we need a fundamental change, bringing to an end the existing system of serious case reviews, and replacing it with a new national learning framework for inquiries into child deaths and cases where children have experienced serious harm. (DfE, 2016: 8)

The government stated that they wanted to end the previous system of SCRs and introduce a two-tier system of nationally led and locally based child safeguarding reviews, the aim of this being to:

> bring greater consistency to public reviews of child protection failures;
>
> improve the speed and quality of reviews, at local and national levels, including through accrediting authors;

make sure that reviews which are commissioned are proportionate to the circumstances of the case they are investigating;

capture and disseminate lessons more effectively, at local and national levels;

make sure lessons inform practice. (DfE, 2016: 7)

The findings of the Wood Review are summarised in the box below.

Summary of Alan Wood's review of Local Safeguarding Children Boards

- Local Safeguarding Children Boards should be abolished and replaced with new flexible local safeguarding arrangements led by three safeguarding partners (local authorities, chief officers of police, and clinical commissioning groups). Those partners will have a duty to make arrangements to work together and with any relevant agencies for the purpose of safeguarding and promoting the welfare of children in their area.
- Safeguarding partners will have to identify and arrange for the review of serious child safeguarding cases which they think raise issues of importance in relation to their area.
- A new, national Child Safeguarding Practice Review Panel has been established. The Panel will commission and publish reviews of child safeguarding cases which it thinks raise issues that are complex or of national importance.
- Clinical commissioning groups and local authorities will have joint responsibility for more general child death reviews, with a potentially wider geographical area for these partnerships allowing them to gain a better understanding of the causes of child deaths.

Implementation of the Wood Review

Having analysed the Wood Review we now move on to explore the system change and leadership challenges implied by the Review and the official response. By October 2019 every local authority area in England had a new child safeguarding architecture in place. More detail than this is very difficult to state with any authority, as *Working Together to Safeguard Children* (HMG, 2018) was in many ways de-regulatory in its effect and is not as prescriptive as was the case with the predecessor *Working Together to Safeguard Children* (HMG, 2015). It is for the 'three partners' in each of the 152 relevant local authority areas to propose how they wish to implement the new arrangements. In some areas the system closely resembles the former LSCB; in other areas the system is radically different.

Each area now has its own Multi-Agency Safeguarding Arrangements (MASA). *Working Together to Safeguard Children* (HMG, 2018) states that each MASA must have a Chief Officer (or a delegated officer) from the local authority, a Chief Officer from the clinical commissioning group (CCG) representing health and someone of similar standing nominated by the Chief Constable of Police. These people are likely to be the Director of Children's Services (DCS), a district commander from the police and a designated professional from the CCG: although this may not be exactly the case in every area. The MASA will have a website – which will contain information on training, learning, policy and procedures that all practitioners should be familiar with for their local area. In summary the aim is to build what Wenger would identify as a new community of practice.

The approach taken in each local area must be assessed by a person or a process who will provide 'independent scrutiny' – a role which, following the Wood Review, has evolved from the previous role of the 'independent chair' of a LSCB, a role which Wood was sceptical of. The three partners must publish a 12-monthly report – which in turn the independent person must scrutinise. This is the element that is supposed to ensure that the system is transparent and open to some form of public accountability. It is noteworthy that one reason that Wood was critical of the independent chair role was that the line of accountability lacked independence – they were formerly appointed by the Chief Executive of the local authority. The new system fails to address Wood's concerns as the independent scrutineer is appointed by the three partners, so again the idea of independence seems seriously compromised.

A central part of the process is that the three partners must identify the 'relevant agencies' that they wish to work with in safeguarding children and young people in the local area. The exact list will vary from locality to locality but will represent a wide range of organisations working with children and young people. Such organisations are mentioned in Chapter Two of *Working Together to Safeguard Children* (HMG, 2018) – the relevant agencies may include prisons, the probation service, early years and childcare organisations and the community and voluntary sector amongst others. This is relevant to the front-line safeguarding practitioners in two ways: as a professional you may actually work for one of the named relevant organisations or you will work in partnership with many of the relevant agencies in your professional role. Either of these places responsibility on practitioners as outlined in *Working Together to Safeguard Children* (HMG, 2018). The 'relevant agencies' in each area will be identified by the three partners and will outline how they will work together in the published arrangements.

There are concerns that some agencies, previously full partners and sitting members of the LSCB, may well feel marginalised by the new arrangements. It is argued here that Wood – and the subsequent State response – was fundamentally flawed. Safeguarding is in essence a multi-professional activity and should not privilege social work, health and police over other practitioners such as early years, probation or housing, for example. As such the Wood reforms are in danger of undermining effective multi-disciplinary working and the considerable achievements of the New Labour *Every Child Matters* era (Frost and Parton, 2009).

Practice point

As a safeguarding professional you should be familiar with your local 'Multi-Agency Safeguarding Arrangements' (MASA), which will have been in place by October 2019, in England.

You should be aware of the new language of safeguarding – as well as MASA. This language includes 'independent scrutiny', 'relevant agencies', 'Child Safeguarding Practice Review' and the '12-monthly report'.

Your local MASA will provide a website which will cover issues such as procedures, policy, training and learning from reviews.

You need to be aware when you are working for a 'relevant agency' or with a 'relevant agency' and be familiar with the local published arrangements in relation to this.

Ensure you are aware of the work of your local safeguarding partnership.

Child Safeguarding Practice Reviews: National and local frameworks

The Wood Review is arguably correct in arguing that the usefulness of Serious Case Reviews (SCRs) has declined over time and their purpose and utility could often be questioned. SCRs were expensive to undertake, often published some considerable time after the relevant events and were frequently criticised for being too repetitive of previous SCRs' findings and recommendations (Brandon et al., 2020). The Wood Review, and later *Working Together to Safeguard Children* (HMG, 2018), introduces a reformed system of learning and case review, with a new language of local and national Child Safeguarding Practice Reviews (CSPRs), which will be crucial in helping to shape the future of safeguarding practice. The first National Review was initiated in April 2019, and addressed the following questions:

Do adolescents in need of state protection from criminal exploitation get the help they need, when they need it?

How can the services designed to keep adolescents safe from criminal exploitation, and the way those services work together, be improved to prevent further harm? (Child Safeguarding Review Panel, 2020: 6)

This new practice review process begins with the statutory duty on the local authority to notify the Child Safeguarding Practice Review Panel if 'a child dies or is seriously harmed' in their area or if they normally reside in the area and are harmed outside of England. This should be notified to the Panel and the other partners within five days of the authority 'becoming aware of the incident'. The local authority must also notify the Secretary of State for Education and Ofsted whenever a looked-after child dies.

The criteria for partnerships carrying out local reviews are that cases:

> raise issues of importance in relation to the area and commission and oversee the review of those cases, where they consider it appropriate for a review to be undertaken. (HMG, 2018: 4:15)

The responsibility for commissioning reviews is devolved to the local MASA. They must decide if it is appropriate to undertake such a review and whether learning can be gained from the process. The reason for carrying out, or not carrying out a review, must be transparent and must be communicated to the relevant family. The MASA must consider whether carrying out a review:

- Highlights the improvements required
- Highlights recurrent themes
- Highlights concerns about how agencies work together
- Reflects the view of the National Panel that a local review may be more appropriate than a national review (see HMG, 2018: 4:18).

Whilst the partners 'must' consider the four bullet points above, *Working Together to Safeguard Children* states that safeguarding partners should also have regard as to whether:

- There is 'cause for concern' about a single agency
- There is no agency involvement and this gives cause for concern
- Where the family have moved around different local authority areas
- Where there are concerns about institutional abuse (HMG, 2018: 4:18).

Where it seems that the criteria may be met, the safeguarding partners should undertake a Rapid Review of the case. This process is about gathering facts, discussing any immediate action required, considering any identified requirements to safeguard children and deciding any next steps and whether a CSPR is required.

A copy of the Rapid Review should be sent to the National Panel, alongside the decision about whether a local review is required. The partners should also inform the Panel, Ofsted and the DfE if they are planning a local review and who the reviewer is.

The local MASA is responsible for commissioning and supervising an independent author for the local child safeguarding reviews. Criteria for the selection of a local reviewer are provided (see HMG, 2018: 4:31). The MASA should negotiate the appropriate methodology with the reviewer, taking into account the Munro Review (Munro, 2011). The review process should make sure that 'practitioners are fully involved in reviews and invited to contribute their perspectives without fear of being blamed for actions they took in good faith' (see HMG, 2018: 4:32). Families should also be invited to contribute and the child or young person should be 'at the centre of the process'.

The final published review should include a summary of 'any recommended improvements' and 'an analysis of any systemic or underlying reasons why actions were taken or not' (HMG, 2018: 4.36). The report should be published, 'unless [the MASA] consider it inappropriate to do so'. If the report is not published the MASA should still publish any suggested improvements that arise from the review. The MASA must also send a copy of the report to the Secretary of State for Education and to Ofsted – at least seven days before publication.

The National Panel also need to consider if a national review is required. The criteria for a national review are that the Panel must consider if the case(s):

- Highlights or may highlight where improvements are required
- Raises issues that may require change to guidance or regulation
- Highlights recurrent themes.

The Panel should also have regard to:

- Significant harm or death to a child educated outside of a school setting
- A child is seriously harmed or dies whilst being looked after or subject to, or recently subject to, a child protection plan
- Where a range of types of abuse is involved
- Where there are issues relating to institutional settings (see HMG, 2018: 4:22).

Where there is to be a national review the National Panel must work with the local MASA (or MASAs) in terms of sharing information, the scope and methodology for the Review and how local partners will be involved in the process. The National Panel have set up a pool of approved reviewers.

The MASA should take into account findings from local and national reviews when considering learning from any review. There should be an auditing and action planning process in relation to implementing any learning from reviews.

━━━━━━━ **Practice point** ━━━━━━━

You should be familiar with the terminology and the processes relating to Local Child Safeguarding Practice Reviews and National Child Safeguarding Practice Reviews.

If you, as a practitioner, are unfortunate enough to be involved in a notifiable case you should be familiar with your organisation's approach to the process of Rapid Review, notifying the DfE and Ofsted and the subsequent review processes. Your senior managers will support you through this process.

You have a professional duty to learn from published local and national review processes. This will be supported through the 'What Works' centre (www.scie.org.UK/children/what-works-centre) who are funded to support the dissemination of learning. This learning will help you meet the expectations of your professional registration.

Understanding 'contextual safeguarding': An emerging direction in safeguarding young people

As we have seen above, *Working Together to Safeguard Children* (HMG, 2018) ushered in a new system of coordinating safeguarding and learning from serious cases – both locally and nationally. In terms of the direct, day-to-day practice these reforms change little for the front-line worker. Chapter One of *Working Together to Safeguard Children* (HMG, 2018) largely reproduces the material on early help, assessment and Section 17 and Section 47 inquiries that practitioners are familiar with from previous editions of *Working Together to Safeguard Children* and which are reflected in local agency procedures.

There is, however, one major change of emphasis in *Working Together to Safeguard Children* (HMG, 2018), reflecting recent changes in the field, and this relates to 'contextual safeguarding'. This has become a concept utilised in order to orientate safeguarding practitioners towards thinking more systemically about issues such as child sexual exploitation, child trafficking, radicalisation, modern slavery and 'county lines' processes (HMG, 2018: 1:33–4). Given the close links between these different forms of contextual abuse it may be the case that the term 'child sexual exploitation' which has had such a high profile in recent years may be displaced as we see how CSE overlaps with many other aspects of contextual safeguarding.

Contextual exploitation refers to abuse or exploitation outside of the family: that is in the 'context' of the community. As a result, assessments and interventions must take into account factors outside of the family – it is a tribute to the robustness of the Assessment Framework (see Horwath and Platt, 2019) that it provides a tool for undertaking this process comprehensively. This issue – of contextual safeguarding – is explored in depth in Chapter 8 of this book.

You should make sure you know how the concept of 'contextual safeguarding' is being deployed, so you can understand your role comprehensively.

When undertaking an assessment and/or implementing a child protection plan, you should think about wider, 'contextual safeguarding' threats to the child or young person coming from outside of the family. The Assessment Framework will assist you in this process.

Working Together to Safeguard Children (2018): A critical overview

This chapter has so far outlined the major policy and practice changes outlined in *Working Together to Safeguard Children* (HMG, 2018). All child welfare and health practitioners are encouraged to think critically about their work and the settings they work in – this section facilitates that process and suggests what some of the issues may be.

▬▬▬▬▬▬▬ **Reflection point** ▬▬▬▬▬▬▬▬▬▬▬▬▬▬

Has *Working Together to Safeguard Children* (HMG, 2018) improved the safeguarding of children and young people in England?

Has the 2018 framework for learning from serious cases been an improvement compared to the previous situation?

The roots of the Alan Wood-based reforms of child safeguarding are difficult to identify – but perhaps lay in the Ofsted judgements in relation to some LSCBs, government criticism of some SCRs (the Hamzah Khan and Daniel Pelka SCRs are examples of this) and a consistent theme that practitioners are somehow responsible when a child dies or is seriously injured. This blame narrative can be seen clearly in the following quote from the then Secretary of State for Education, Michael Gove:

I want to talk about child protection. Specifically, how we care for the most vulnerable children – those at risk of neglect or abuse – those who come into the care of others because their families cannot care for them. And I want to begin with an admission. The state is currently failing in its duty to keep our children safe. (Michael Gove, Secretary of State, 16 November 2012)

Gove is clearly deploying a blame narrative here and later also refers to 'a failure of leadership'. This is a damaging narrative suggesting that the safeguarding system is 'failing' and is deeply embedded in political and media accounts. As we have mentioned, it sometimes unites the political right (Michael Gove, for example) and the political left (see Featherstone et al., 2014, for example). Practitioners working in the system know how many children are effectively protected and this positive position tends to be upheld by international statistical analysis (see Pritchard and Williams, 2009, for example, and current trends in the reduction in the rate of child deaths, NSPCC, 2018).

The position taken in this book is against this blame culture and argues it is both negative and damaging – whether coming from the political right or left. LSCBs had succeeded in promoting a multi-agency culture, training large numbers of staff, responding to shared safeguarding challenges, such as child sexual exploitation (CSE) and ensuring that policy and procedures are effectively shared and owned. If we reflect carefully then it is actually counter-intuitive that a range of qualified and experienced practitioners would come together in order to do their best for children and somehow fail. When a child dies it is rarely, if ever, the fault of a professional, a point argued by Professor Eileen Munro (2005, 2011) and such accusations also tend to take the blame away from the often violent men who are usually the perpetrators. The Wood Review also misinterprets the data gathered by the Local Government Association by Baginsky and Holmes (2015). They indeed argued that:

> No evidence was found to support notions of structural or procedural reform to LSCBs; and indeed any reform activity would first require the establishment of shared and realistic expectations of LSCBs together with recognition of the many contextual pressures placed upon them. (2015: 8)

The dangers of the nationally diverse system proposed by Wood and now implemented are apparent:

- Cross-authority communication is more difficult – in the previous system this took place between LSCB chair and LSCB chair, or LSCB manager and LSCB manager. It is complex to find out who to communicate with in the new architecture.
- Professional pre-qualifying training is more difficult. Pre-*Working Together to Safeguard Children* (HMG, 2018) a trainer/lecturer would inform all students that the LSCB would provide information on policy, procedures and training, for example. Post-*Working Together to Safeguard Children* there is no shared organisational structure which can be clearly outlined to emergent practitioners.

In contrast, the abolition of the SCR system seems to be a step forward. As argued earlier, the system seems to have become expensive and repetitive – the new approach through Child Safeguarding Practice Reviews will hopefully re-invigorate the process and create new learning opportunities. One concern here is the inclusion of the word 'practice' in the title – this may lead to the blaming process rather than a focus on the challenges of emergent forms of abuse (child criminal exploitation, for example) where the focus should be on the issue rather than practice as such. It is unclear at the time of writing how the system of national reviews will evolve – just how frequent and how high profile they will be is something that will only emerge over time, following the publication of the first review in 2020 (Child Safeguarding Review Panel, 2020).

Multi-disciplinary working in practice

The underpinning logic of *Working Together to Safeguard Children* is aimed at enhancing day-to-day practice, policy work and both local and national learning from Child Safeguarding Practice Reviews. It is based in an assumption that children and young people are more effectively safeguarded when practitioners work together effectively. Brandon et al. conclude as follows in relation to Serious Case Reviews and multi-disciplinary working:

- The language we use to talk about children's circumstances can both support and hinder effective safeguarding.
- Fragmentation of services, with different front-line providers within the same agency, can lead to silo-working within as well as between agencies.
- Clear multi-agency plans at both child in need and child protection levels are central to effective working. (2020: 20)

In summary, high quality multi-disciplinary working should avoid:

1 A lack of information sharing (see the Baby Peter SCR, for example)
2 Damaging organisational conflicts and disputes (see the Cleveland inquiry)
3 A lack of focus on the child's world and their journey (see the Victoria Climbié report).

It follows then that effective multi-disciplinary working achieves the opposite of the negatives uncovered by SCRs: we should work towards a holistic, child-centred approach drawing on shared professional goals and based on agreed organisational policy and procedure.

Conclusion

This chapter has aimed to:

- Utilise the theoretical model of 'communities of practice' to reach a critical assessment of multi-disciplinary working
- Explore the current system of organising and planning the safeguarding system, utilising the English example
- Critically assess the current system for enhancing multi-disciplinary working.

This chapter has outlined and provided a critical analysis of the current system of safeguarding in England. It has been argued that effective multi-disciplinary working is a cornerstone of safeguarding children, and that this can be embedded through the utilisation of a communities of practice model. It has also been argued that the current system is actually working relatively well to safeguard children and the political utilisation of a blame culture is both damaging and unhelpful.

Recommended reading

Etienne Wenger, *Communities of Practice* (1999)

> Wenger's book has 'classic' status and has been utilised in the public, community, voluntary and private sectors alike as a model for improving 'working together'. The theoretical model can be applied practically in safeguarding as well as in other settings. For more detail and applications see https://wenger-trayner.com/introduction-to-communities-of-practice/ (accessed 16 February 2020).

HMG, *Working Together to Safeguard Children* (2018)

> This is the English model for achieving effective multi-disciplinary work in the safeguarding world. The text has been through many iterations, reflecting the politics of the day and recent developments in safeguarding. Whilst elements of the text are ideologically driven, particularly the de-regulation of local partnerships, the practice element is well tested and evidence-based. Essential reading for all England-based practitioners.

Jan Horwath and Dendy Platt, *The Child's World* (2019)

> Currently in its third edition this is the 'highway code' for children's safeguarding work. The book contains a wide range of expertly authored chapters which provide sound practice experience, based in theory and research: particularly strong in relation to assessment skills.

3

UNDERSTANDING CHILD ABUSE AND CHILD PROTECTION

CONTENTS

The aims of this chapter are to:

- Define and understand what we mean by key terms and concepts
- Explore the incidence of child abuse and neglect
- Present and analyse legal and regulatory frameworks
- Examine multi-professional responses to child abuse and neglect
- Explain different theoretical approaches to understanding child abuse

Introduction

This chapter attempts to bring together frameworks for understanding child abuse and child protection. The chapter extends one of the key arguments of the book relating to the social construction of child abuse and the impact of these contested understandings on actual safeguarding practice. The chapter draws on international sources to work towards a global perspective on child protection issues. The following Chapter 4 applies some of these theories to two specific in-depth case studies: one relating to abuse by a celebrity, Jimmy Savile, and one in relation to institutional abuse.

What is child abuse?

One of the key assumptions of this book is that our understanding of child abuse and our collective responses to it are socially constructed. That is, as discussed earlier, there is no fixed, 'natural' or universally agreed phenomenon that we can define as child abuse: the phenomenon of child abuse varies according to the historical time it takes place and the location it occurs in. This argument is developed and the implications of this formulation are taken further throughout the chapter.

As we argued in Chapter 1, child abuse varies across time and this can be illustrated by exploring social history. It has also been argued earlier that an understanding of social history enhances our grasp of contemporary practice. In Victorian England, for example, children were used to undertake various dangerous tasks in factories, on farms and in such work as cleaning chimneys (Kirby, 2003). What was then the 'norm' we would now regard as dangerous and abusive, or indeed we would now name it as 'modern slavery'. If you ask people born in the UK during the 1950s or before, they may well remember children being caned in school settings (Middleton, 2008): a social practice that would involve the police if it were to happen in the twenty-first century. It can be seen, therefore, that abuse and our responses to it vary across time, even across relatively short historical periods.

Child abuse also varies across space, or by geography. For example, on a recent visit to India the author witnessed a girl, perhaps seven years of age, working outside in the searing heat, chipping large boulders into smaller chips: this would be illegal and her employer would be arrested if this occurred in the United Kingdom.

Reflection point

If you have travelled abroad think about the lives of children in different cultures.

In southern Mediterranean cultures (Spain and Italy, for example) you may notice that the culture is more child-centred with many play areas and children being accepted in restaurants late at night. How does this compare and contrast with where you live or practise?

What are the implications for attitudes to childhood and for safeguarding?

See Woolcock (2016) for ways of measuring childhood across the globe.

How we understand child abuse today is defined by a series of complex social practices, narratives and laws which generate our, contemporary, understandings of abuse: these can change rapidly as was seen in the first decade of the twenty-first century in the United Kingdom. At the start of this century, in 2000, the phrase child sexual exploitation (CSE) was rarely used and the phenomenon was not really understood. By 2010 this situation had changed and CSE went on to become identified as a major challenge for practitioners and was subject to extensive media and political attention (see Chapter 7 for an in-depth discussion of this). This provides a graphic example of how safeguarding itself – and our understanding and response to it – change over a relatively short time. It also illustrates how important concepts are: it was the emergent concept of 'child sexual exploitation' that changed perceptions and displaced 'child prostitution' as a phrase that, in turn, had generated punitive and blaming forms of response to young people.

Our contemporary understanding is constructed by a complex interplay of law, guidance, managerial and inspectorial expectations, political and media attitudes and professional practice, values and skills. These and many other factors construct contemporary safeguarding policies and practices in relation to children and young people. The authors of the triennial review of Serious Case Reviews highlighted complexity as a key theme of their analysis:

As we looked into the reviews of children affected by serious and fatal child maltreatment between 2014 and 2017, we, too, were struck by the complexity of the lives of these children and families, and the challenges – at times quite overwhelming – faced by the practitioners seeking to support them in such complexity. (Brandon et al., 2020: 23)

This complexity makes measurement of the extent of abuse complicated as well: when the media report an increase in child sexual exploitation, for example, it may well be there has not been any such increase but rather a change of practice awareness of, and the definition of, that particular social problem and that this has led to the perception of an increase.

Given this complex construction of child abuse what can we learn about the extent of child abuse and the need for effective safeguarding?

Child abuse: Definitions and incidence

Whilst it remains true that responses to child abuse vary geographically this is perhaps less so in recent decades where globalisation has had an impact and helped to develop internationally shared understandings of child abuse. The United Nations (UN), the United Nations International Children's Emergency Fund (UNICEF), the World Health Organization (WHO) and many other non-governmental organisations (NGOs) have developed global databases, definitions and analyses of child abuse. Using their lead, we can move towards understanding child abuse as a global issue and concern.

A useful starting point is the *United Nations Convention on the Rights of the Child* (UNCRC). The Convention, which came into force in 1992, has been ratified by all members of the United Nations, with the notable exception of the USA. The Convention forms the basis for many different child and young person related forms of legislation around the world. Whilst all sections of the UN Convention are relevant to the well-being of children and young people, amongst the specific sections relating to child abuse and safeguarding is Article 19, outlined as follows:

19.1 States Parties shall take all appropriate legislative, administrative, social and educational measures to protect the child from all forms of physical or mental violence, injury or abuse, neglect or negligent treatment, maltreatment or exploitation, including sexual abuse, while in the care of parent(s), legal guardian(s) or any other person who has the care of the child.

19.2 Such protective measures should, as appropriate, include effective procedures for the establishment of social programmes to provide necessary support for the child and for those who have the care of the child, as well as for other forms of prevention and for identification, reporting, referral, investigation, treatment and follow-up.

The WHO have attempted to measure and provide data about the extent of child abuse around the world. They define child maltreatment as follows:

Child maltreatment is the abuse and neglect of people under 18 years of age. It includes all forms of physical and/or emotional ill-treatment, sexual abuse, neglect or negligent treatment or commercial or other exploitation, resulting in actual or potential harm to the child's health, survival, development or dignity in the context of a relationship of responsibility, trust or power. Four types of child maltreatment are generally recognized: physical abuse, sexual abuse, psychological (or emotional or mental) abuse, and neglect. (http://apps.who.int/violence-info/child-maltreatment, accessed 17 February 2020)

To underpin this work the WHO have estimated the global percentage of children and young people who have experienced various forms of abuse, as outlined in Table 3.1.

Table 3.1 Global lifetime prevalence of child maltreatment (WHO, 2014)

Type of abuse	Percentage of child population
Psychological abuse	36
Physical abuse	23
Sexually abused girls	18
Sexually abused boys	8
Neglect	16

We can see that child abuse is an extensive social problem and that there is an emerging global consensus around the importance of child safeguarding; however, implementation, and in particular, the provision of services through the social programmes identified by the UN, varies considerably around the world.

The NSPCC, in the UK, produce an annual publication addressing the question 'how safe are our children?' For example, their extensive reports make it clear that the five-year annual average child homicide rates in England, Northern Ireland and Scotland have declined over the past decade (NSPCC, 2018: 20). The NSPCC utilise an innovative self-report method asking people aged 18–24 to assess if they have been abused during their childhood. In terms of severe physical maltreatment 11.5% reported that they had experienced this. In relation to contact sexual abuse 11.3% reported this – although the figure was much higher amongst females (17.8%) as opposed to males (5.1%). Severe neglect by a parent is also more prevalent amongst females (11%) than males (7%), giving a rate of 9% across the whole sample. Severe maltreatment by a parent was reported by 14.5% (11.6% male, 17.5% female). This gives a total of 21.3% reporting some abuse during childhood – 30.6% of females and 20.3% of males. In summary we can see that over one-fifth of the population report being abused during their childhood, rising to almost one-third of all females.

We can see, therefore, that child abuse is a widespread social problem, whether measured globally or in an advanced Western society. Child abuse is not spread evenly amongst population groups of course: it can be seen in Table 3.1 that girls are more likely to be subject to sexual abuse, for example. It is also the case that children with disabilities may be more vulnerable to abuse:

> Disabled children and young people are three times more likely to be abused or neglected than other children and young people. Children who are at particular risk include those with learning difficulties/disabilities, speech and language difficulties, health related conditions and deaf children. (Shaw, 2016: 3)

It is crucial for such groups of children and young people that we do what we can to prevent abuse and neglect: safeguarding should always be underpinned by prevention. As the abuse of children and young people is a major global challenge it is also a challenge that demands a global policy framework. These social and preventative programmes can draw upon the INSPIRE programme designed by the WHO. The nine elements of this programme are explained in the box below.

INSPIRE programme, World Health Organization

Societies should:

- create safe, sustainable and nurturing family environments, and provide specialized help and support for families at risk of violence;
- modify unsafe environments through physical changes;
- reduce risk factors in public spaces (e.g. schools, places where young people gather) to reduce the threat of violence;
- address gender inequities in relationships, the home, school, the workplace;
- change the cultural attitudes and practices that support the use of violence;
- ensure legal frameworks prohibit all forms of violence against children and limit youth access to harmful products, such as alcohol and firearms;
- provide access to quality response services for children affected by violence;
- eliminate the cultural, social and economic inequalities that contribute to violence, close the wealth gap and ensure equitable access to goods, services and opportunities;
- coordinate the actions of the multiple sectors that have a role to play in preventing and responding to violence against children.

The INSPIRE programme is both aspirational and inspirational and provides a useful programme for potential change and progress. The prevention of child abuse should be prioritised internationally and should also underpin more targeted child protection approaches. This issue is pursued further in the concluding chapter of this book.

━━━━━━━━━━ **Reflection point** ━━━━━━━━━━

What do you think should be prioritised, in policy terms, in order to reduce and prevent child abuse in your nation state?

Legal frameworks

One of the ways that our understanding of child abuse is socially constructed is through legal frameworks: unsurprisingly these too vary historically and geographically. One way of understanding the law is through the lens of the relationship between the State and the household. Of course, contextual abuse is different and involves localities and can be trans-national. The State/household issue is a complex one and arguably lies at the heart of the debates and controversies about child abuse: it is one reason why professional roles in relation to protecting children are always complex and demanding and it is why child protection practice is never straightforward. Some political perspectives on safeguarding, which can be defined as paternalistic and/or interventionist, support extensive State intervention in the family if this works to protect children (see Fox-Harding, 2014, who provides a useful framework for understanding these issues). Where this is the case we would expect to find higher numbers of children subject to legal processes and perhaps being looked after by the State. Other political perspectives, which can be defined as non-interventionist or pro-family, would only defend State intervention in the most extreme of circumstances and as a result there may be fewer children subject to proceedings or looked after by the State. These different perspectives are always in tension and can change and develop very quickly – after a well-publicised child abuse death, for example, the rate of care proceedings may well increase (Parton, 2017).

The tension between these interventionist and non-interventionist stances can be seen in the UN Charter and are embedded within the English Children Act 1989, for example. The Children Act assumes non-intervention in the family (for example, see Section 1 of the Act) and provides for services to support families in caring for their own children, in Section 17 of the Act, for example. But the Act also has interventionist elements (Section 40 and Section 47), aimed at protecting and looking after children who have suffered, or may suffer, from 'significant harm'. There is an inherent tension between these interventionist and non-interventionist perspectives which is played out in children's social care offices and family courts throughout the country, and in different forms across the world. The mobilisation of this tension and how it works out depends on demanding and nuanced professional judgements: it is why child protection is always complex and often is in the public eye. To address these complexities requires high level professional skills and forms of knowledge, which are explored in Chapter 9 of this book. The recognition of these complexities should also make us wary of the blame culture often adopted by the media and politicians in relation to child abuse deaths or scandals, which were discussed in Chapter 2 of this book.

Understanding abuse

There are many ways of understanding child abuse and neglect: each theory is worthy of a book in itself and here we can only summarise some of these briefly. Suggestions for further, in-depth reading are provided at the end of the chapter.

Different practitioners and academics hold contrasting explanations of the phenomenon of child abuse and how we should respond to it as safeguarding practitioners. Below we attempt to explain, as independently as possible, some of these schools of thought – exploring elements of their respective strengths and weaknesses.

Behavioural explanations

The behaviourist school uses the lens of human behaviour and examines how this behaviour is formed and reformed to understand the underpinnings of child abuse. A behavioural approach explores the determinants of human behaviour and behaviourists often root this in forms of human nature, for example, seeing the attachment between mother and child as a natural form of behaviour and a deviation from this as something that is 'dysfunctional' and can be changed and reformed. Understandings of behaviourism have roots in experiments, on both humans and animals, that aim to show that behaviour can be changed in response to rewards and punishments: a process known as 'operant conditioning'. B.F. Skinner, perhaps the most influential behaviourist, writes that:

> it is in the nature of an experimental analysis of human behaviour that it should strip away the functions previously assigned to a free or autonomous person and transfer them one by one to the controlling environment. (1971: 198)

The human being then is seen as a bundle of behaviours – there is no need to focus on the underlying or unconscious elements of these behaviours, simply on the stimulus and the response. There are many criticisms that can be made of behaviourism. It can be argued that this approach reduces human beings to mere stimuli and related responses – and thus underplays the complexity of human responses. It also tends to ignore the wider social context in which human beings exist and thus would struggle to explain social class or ethnic differences, for example.

Ecological explanations

A significant amount of child safeguarding practice and thinking is rooted in differing forms of ecological thinking – that is, that the child and their family are located in a nest of systems that exist at different levels. This theory often draws on the work of Urie Bronfenbrenner (1979), whose work has influenced the assessment triangle which is discussed in Chapter 5 of this book. Bronfenbrenner's systems begin with those closest to the child: the micro system, which is the immediate environment of the child, the family or household that the child lives in. The meso system is the wider system of interaction between the home and, say, the school or day care setting. The exo system is wider again – focused on the community, or the parent's workplace, for example. The macro system is the wider social, economic and political context that influences childhood experiences in the broadest sense. Some models of Bronfenbrenner's work include the chrono system – which addresses one of the themes of this book, change over a period of time. A clear advantage of the ecological approach is that it is multi-levelled, it does not simply focus on the social or the individual but can locate safeguarding issues within a flexible, multi-level model. This can be used by the professional to work out where safeguarding issues are located: for example, in parenting styles within the household, or more widely, in the social policies of the government that help to form childhood.

Feminist explanations

Feminists see gender and gender inequality as fundamental to understanding society in general, and to understanding child abuse more specifically. A feminist analysis, which has informed much of this book, sees child abuse as part of the wider abuse of male power. This analysis is particularly applicable to child sexual abuse where the most common form is abuse of females by males: child sexual exploitation would be a powerful example of this. Domestic abuse, and the murder of female partners by males in household settings, provide further graphic examples of how gender helps explain safeguarding issues. Many of the leading scholars in the field of child abuse have been feminists: Linda Gordon and Liz Kelly are just two examples whose worked is quoted throughout this book. The feminist analysis of neglect and physical abuse is rather more complex: most perpetrators of these forms of abuse are female. This relates to women being the main caregivers and also being more likely to experience poverty. In order for feminist theories to be applicable in child abuse we also need to take into account age and generation which represents another form of power differential in society. Judith Ennew takes ethnicity, wealth, gender and generation into account in her powerful study of child sexual exploitation, a form of analysis which has become known as 'intersectionality' (Crenshaw, 1990; Davis, 2008).

Psychological explanations

There are many schools of psychological explanation which can be applied to child abuse. Behaviourism as discussed earlier is a form of psychology – there are also schools of cognitive, social and forensic psychology which could be applied to our understanding of child abuse. There are psychoanalytic schools, which may draw on Freud and Jung, and focus on early childhood experiences and the role of the unconscious. What these approaches have in common is a focus on the individual and their psychological make-up: although to complicate matters there are also forms of social psychology, such approaches are often described as psycho-social. For some psychological schools a male who has a poor experience of mothering, may grow up to have a negative view of women, and be involved in abusing girls or women as he gets older. The roots of abuse are therefore to be found in the psychological development of the individual, albeit in a social context. Attachment theory drawing on the psychological work of John Bowlby and colleagues has been particularly influential in relation to safeguarding. The early work of Bowlby focused on early attachment between mother and child, but recent developments are more flexible and multi-faceted (Harlow, 2019). Depending on the school of psychology, treatment for disorders could be a talking therapy, such as psychoanalysis or cognitive behavioural therapy (CBT), or may involve medication. Social psychology may overlap more with systems theory and feminist explanations, explored in this chapter, and may embrace social change to address issues of child protection.

Social structural explanations

A school of child protection scholars have adopted social structural explanations of child abuse. Such thinking draws on radical social theory – influenced by Marxism and related schools of thought. This approach places social class, poverty and inequality at the heart of the analysis (Bywaters, 2013). These scholars argue that parenting is more difficult in poverty and that this is one reason why the majority of families subject to child protection interventions are poor families. These families are also more visible to social agencies as they are dependent on the State for many aspects of their lives – perhaps including income support, education, health and housing. This approach would also look at global inequalities to explain differing patterns of abuse across the world (Marre and Briggs, 2009)

The challenge of social structural explanations is that even if one is sympathetic to them, it is difficult to translate this form of explanation to actual practice with a given family. This has been attempted, however, for example by Corrigan and Leonard (1978) and more recently by Featherstone and colleagues (2018). For social structural theorists the causes and impact of safeguarding require fundamental social change.

Systems-based explanations

There are many systems theorists in the field of child protection. These theories relate to two different systems: family systems and organisational systems. The focus is on the system rather than on the individual. Systems theory of the family sees families working as a system, with sub-systems within the household. For example, two parents with three children form a system, but within this the sibling group may form a sub-system. When families work well, these systems can be seen as functioning efficiently: when not they are described as dysfunctional. A school of family therapy can be used to explore when things are not working well: the therapist looks at how the systems are working and suggests ways that the operation and interactions between the systems could be changed. Bowen was a leading proponent of this approach, as outlined below:

> Bowen's focus was on patterns that develop in families in order to defuse anxiety. A key generator of anxiety in families is the perception of either too much closeness or too great a distance in a relationship: The degree of anxiety in any one family will be determined by the current levels of external stress and the sensitivities to particular themes that have been transmitted down the generations. If family members do not have the capacity to think through their responses to relationship dilemmas, but rather react anxiously to perceived emotional demands, a state of chronic anxiety or reactivity may be set in place. (Brown, 1999: 94)

Eileen Munro (2005) is amongst the leading advocates of systems theory as a method of understanding how the child protection system works. The approach shares much with the systems approach to families – seeing the child protection system as one which consists of a number of interlocking systems. It follows that when things go wrong in the safeguarding system the focus should be on the working of the system rather than the individual:

> A system-centred approach looks for causal explanation of error in all parts of the system, not just within the individual … the human operator is only one factor, the final outcome is the product of the interaction of the individual with the rest of the system. (Munro, 2005: 534)

This quote provides a useful rejoinder to the blame culture discussed and criticised in Chapter 2 of this book.

A pragmatic approach?

Readers of this book will have some sympathy – and no doubt some differences – with the perspectives outlined in the discussion above. In reality most practitioners will take a pragmatic, or eclectic, approach to their safeguarding work. This will often depend on the actual context you work in and the purpose of your organisation. What does this mean in practice? The professional may take a social structural approach to understanding their work: they will probably be aware that many of their service users are poor, unemployed and perhaps dependent on food banks to survive. The same professional may well take an ecological approach to working with a specific child: perhaps the school system is not working well for the child. There may also be a poor relationship between the child and a parent – where some sort of psycho-social approach would be helpful. A professional should not be embarrassed by taking such a pragmatic approach; as long as the approach is thoughtful and reflective, it may well be appropriate to the situation that the professional is seeking to understand and respond to.

Reflection point

Do you have a theory – it may be mentioned above – which influences the way you think about and practise in relation to safeguarding?

Which approach is best suited to the stated aims and purpose of your organisation?

Reflect on the strengths and weaknesses of any theory you prefer.

Responding to child abuse

Having identified potential conceptual and legal frameworks for understanding the abuse of children we now move on to explore the nature of professional responses. Again, rehearsing a core theme of this book, these responses are socially constructed: there is no one 'technically correct' manner of responding to child abuse, only socially specific and situational responses which are mandated at a given time, in any given society. The link between a specific situation and a response to it is always complex and is often potentially both controversial and contested.

Table 3.2 presents a framework for analysing how different perspectives generate different responses.

Table 3.2 Different perspectives on child abuse

Child protection orientation	Underpinning theory	Legal mandates	Research findings	Forms of practice	Potential challenges
A strong State approach	The State has a responsibility to protect children from abuse in the family and/or the community	UN Convention on the Rights of the Child – rights to protection S.47 Children Act 1989 (England)	Findings of Serious Case Reviews/Child Safeguarding Practice Reviews	The State should act with authority and swiftly to ensure children are as effectively protected as possible	The State is too authoritative, with the rights of families undermined and too many children are entering the care system
Pro-family/ parent-focused	Children are usually best cared for within the family. Poor families face inequalities for which they should not be penalised by losing their children	UN Convention on the Rights of the Child – rights to protection	Research findings on the impact of poverty on families (Bywaters et al., 2016b), the family support literature and research challenging the child protection system (Featherstone et al., 2018)	An emphasis on challenging inequalities and providing supportive services for families	Children are left at home in dangerous situations and *in extremis* may die
Child-centred	Practitioners should have a clear focus on the child as they are powerless in the household and in need of protection	UN Convention on the Rights of the Child – rights to participation	The mainstream literature of being child-centred – Race and O'Keefe (2017) and *Working Together to Safeguard Children* (HMG, 2018)	Exploring the needs of the child and using practice techniques which listen to them and enable them to participate	The focus on the child means that the needs of the family, particularly arising from inequalities, are not addressed

We can see in Table 3.2 that different orientations are possible within different organisational settings and under the broad banner of safeguarding – e.g. exploring a strong State response, a pro-family approach and a child-centred approach (see Parton, 2017, for further analysis). All these responses can be argued to have an ethical underpinning and a basis in law. Different research evidence can be provided to back up these responses: this, once again, is why safeguarding is a complex activity. Each approach has strengths but also contain within them many challenges and potential downsides. Part of being a professional is reflecting on your values, aligning these with professional standards and balancing this against legal frameworks and political and economic contexts. One aim of this book is to facilitate the reflective professional in reaching their own position on these complex questions.

Refection point

Consider the three different approaches outlined above: a strong State response, a pro-family approach and a child-centred approach.

Is there one approach that you are most sympathetic with?

Why is this the case?

Conclusion

This chapter has aimed to:

- Define and understand what we mean by key terms and concepts
- Explore the incidence of child abuse and neglect
- Present and analyse legal and regulatory frameworks
- Examine multi-professional responses to child abuse and neglect
- Explain different theoretical approaches to understanding child abuse.

Each reader will respond differently to the complex and demanding issues explored in this chapter. We have seen that abuse is complex, global and extensive and takes many diverse forms. The professional needs to be aware of the challenges of recognising and responding to abuse. Having established these challenges and complexities the book now moves to provide two case studies, on celebrity abuse and institutional abuse, which provide in-depth analysis with some transferable learning.

Recommended reading

NSPCC, *How Safe are our Children?* (annual)

A comprehensive annual report which measures the prevalence of child abuse and changes over recent years. This is an invaluable source book that ensures that debates are underpinned by facts and figures. A new version is published each year and is available on the NSPCC website.

United Nations Convention on the Rights of the Child (UNCRC)

The universal starting point for understanding child abuse and safeguarding policies and practices. The Convention has provided an effective benchmark for building safeguarding systems around the world, whilst attempting to ensure that children's rights are both promoted and protected.

Paul Bywaters and colleagues, *The Relationship between Poverty, Child Abuse and Neglect: An Evidence Review* (2016b)

Here, and elsewhere, Bywaters and colleagues provide an empirical basis for understanding the relationship between poverty, inequality and child protection.

Joanna Nicholas, *Practical Guide to Child Protection* (2015)

This is a readable, applied and practical book that helps us understand and respond to child abuse effectively and in a child-centred manner. A very useful read for students and newly qualified practitioners.

4

EXPLORING TWO CASE STUDIES: ABUSE BY CELEBRITIES AND ABUSE IN INSTITUTIONS

CONTENTS

The aims of this chapter are to:

- Explore the phenomenon of abuse by celebrities: developing the concept of 'accumulated celebrity abuse'
- Explore abuse of children and young people in institutional settings
- Apply learning from these settings to our theoretical and practical understanding of child abuse

Introduction

To facilitate our understanding and further develop the themes discussed in Chapter 3 we explore two specific case studies: the first one looking at the phenomenon of abuse by 'celebrities', using the former English DJ and television presenter Jimmy Savile as an example, and the other exploring abuse in institutional settings. Whilst these are focused and specific, the learning from these case studies is transferable to other situations where child abuse may occur: primarily how the abuse of power actually happens in different settings and outside of the household. In order to discuss these accurately it is necessary to provide some graphic detail of the assaults, which the reader should bear in mind prior to reading.

Case study one: Understanding 'celebrity' abuse – a case study of Jimmy Savile

This section of the book provides a case study of what can be conceptualised as 'accumulated celebrity abuse'. The case study is chosen as it illustrates a fundamental issue in understanding child abuse: that is that child abuse is ultimately an abuse of power. It is argued here that abuse by celebrities is a particular example of the abuse of power. The analysis draws mainly on the report provided by Dame Janet Smith entitled *The Jimmy Savile Investigation Report* (2016a), and is informed by a sister report into the abuse carried out by TV presenter Stuart Hall (2016b) at the British Broadcasting Corporation (BBC).

The case study commences with a wider analysis of the BBC, popular culture and the celebrity DJ during the period that Jimmy Savile was a high-profile celebrity (Greer and McLaughlin, 2013). Having established this wider context the analysis then moves on to explore the link between Savile, the BBC and sexual abuse. It is argued that a new concept – that of 'accumulated celebrity power' – is useful in explaining a form of abuse that has specific features and requires an informed public policy response. A framework used to explain the impact of child sexual abuse, drawing on Finkelhor and Browne's (1985) analysis, is used to explain the impact of sexual abuse on victims.

The initial impression in reading the Smith report about Jimmy Savile's sexual abuse within the BBC setting is one of shock. The reader is shocked about the extent of the abuse, the period of time over which the abuse took place and the brutality of the sexual attacks. It is important to remain professional when we come across disturbing information, but it is also important that we remain both human and humane in our responses. This case study moves on to analyse the key issues that emerge from the report around Savile's sexual crimes utilising the following themes:

1   The abuse of power
2   The role of the celebrity
3   The silence of the victims
4   The institutional nature of the abuse.

First of all, in order to understand the wider context, we explore the more general social and organisational environment in which the abuse took place.

The 1960s: Sex, power and culture at the BBC

The United Kingdom underwent a period of dramatic social change in the early 1960s – popular culture was central to this change (Seabrook, 2006). Popular culture itself was transformed in the short period between 1960 and 1965. This change was led by the pop group The Beatles and linked to shifting social attitudes to sexuality, fashion, contraception and drug use, to name just a few aspects of the social change of the period (Gould, 2007).

The BBC existed in a contradictory space during this period. In many ways it was the carrier of traditional values: well-spoken newsreaders, Saturday night family entertainment and the playing of the National Anthem at the end of broadcasting all being emblematic of this traditional role as the representative of the British Empire that had only recently faded. In contrast to this traditional message was an emergent culture – it was young, brash and sometimes anti-establishment (Seabrook, 2006). The BBC straddled this difficult cultural space.

In order to operate effectively in the new environment the emerging DJs needed big personalities. Jimmy Savile and Kenny Everett represented the most eccentric – making the 'old school' DJs look old-fashioned and not part of the new zeitgeist. The genre was also gendered – some female voices were to be heard, including female DJs such as Annie Nightingale and Liz Kershaw – but these women were marginalised. The DJ was predominantly male and eccentric (Snow, 1987). This radio DJ culture existed in a close relationship with TV and particularly with *Top of the Pops* – a programme which commenced in 1964 and was fronted by many of the Radio One personality DJs (Fryer, 1997).

The popular music celebrity DJ was not, however, constrained to presenting popular music programmes: they presented quiz shows, variety shows and the novelty programmes that Savile became famous for, family TV programmes such as *Jim'll Fix It* and *Savile's Travels*. This extended, in a way that now seems supremely ironic in hindsight, to issues such as child safety in the home:

> Between October and December 1981 at 6.30 p.m. on Sunday evenings on BBC 1, ten 10-minute programmes about childhood accidents were televised. The series was called 'Play it safe' and was introduced by Jimmy Savile. (Colver et al., 1982: 1178)

These people, usually male, accumulate fame, money and celebrity – a process that we conceptualise in this book as 'accumulated celebrity power' – which in the case of Savile was utilised to abuse and sexually assault a wide range of people. His victims included children, young people and adults, males and females (Smith, 2016a).

Sexual abuse: Savile and the abuse of power at the BBC

Having explored the wider context of the BBC and the role of celebrity and power, we move on more specifically to explore the nature of sexual abuse crimes and understand them as an undesirable social phenomenon, built on 'accumulated celebrity power'.

The abuse of power

The world's leading authority on child abuse, David Finkelhor, wrote that child abuse gravitates towards the point of the 'greatest power differential' (1984: 18). This power differential is seen, for example, in intra-familial abuse between a child and a father. In this context one is struck in reading the Smith report by the power that accumulates around 'celebrity'. This power arises from 'fame', 'networks', the 'gaze' of the camera and from celebrity as a 'magnetic' attraction for many members of the public. There is therefore a clear connection between power and celebrity – it is argued here that celebrity magnifies the power that is referred to by Finkelhor (see also Ennew, 1986). In Savile's case, largely due to perceptions that he was active in charity and voluntary work, this power was validated by the Church and State (Smith, 2016a: 772) – Savile received a Papal award and was knighted by the Queen to become Sir Jimmy Savile. The celebrity then accumulates a magnified form of power which is validated by powerful external sources.

Underpinning child sexual abuse, of course, is the issue of gender. Whilst the majority of Savile's victims at the BBC were female (57 victims), some were male (15 victims).

Savile's abuse was primarily the abuse of male power over females and often over female children. The abuse took place in what the Smith report refers to as the 'testosterone fuelled environment' of *Top of the Pops*. The 'gaze' of *Top of the Pops* was predominantly male and many of the female BBC employees report being routinely sexually harassed in their work roles: it is impossible to envisage a female celebrity abusing on the scale of Savile's case. We need therefore to link the power of celebrity to male power in society more generally.

The role of 'celebrity' in sexual abuse

Savile deployed his celebrity power to abuse people – as we have seen this included children and adults, male and female, alike. 'Grooming' is a key concept in sexual abuse in general and in understanding Savile's method in particular. As the Smith report notes, it would be hard to imagine a better designed grooming tool than programmes such as *Savile's Travels* and *Jim'll Fix It*. Both portrayed Savile as the hero – the person able to provide a treat and deliver a wish-fulfilment for the child. These mechanisms allowed him to separate the child from parents that may otherwise have protected the child: again this is a familiar grooming technique. Savile placed himself as the generous provider and the child as a grateful recipient. The Smith report is cynical about this and suggests that Savile actually did little of the practical work himself. Thus, the power differentials present in all adult/child relationships are exaggerated in the Savile context as the programmes provide a mechanism and environment for abusive practices to operate: Savile fundamentally betrays the trust of the victim. Finkelhor and Browne refer to this dynamic in sexual abuse as:

> *Betrayal* … the dynamic by which children discover that someone on whom they were vitally dependent has caused them harm. This may occur in a variety of ways in a molestation experience. (Finkelhor and Browne, 1985: 2)

Savile's grooming technique was in fact short and brutal (Smith, 2016a: 285, for example). He often abused without preliminaries or even conversation. His grooming technique was built around enabling access – to tickets, events or premises: once this access was enabled this was his gateway to sexual abuse. The abuse was then sudden, brutal and direct – it is a strong contrast to that outlined in the sister report (Smith, 2016b) where Stuart Hall used champagne, for example, as part of a more extended and 'subtle' abuse technique (Smith, 2016b: 72). One is struck in reading the Smith report how similar many of the survivor accounts are in outlining Savile's mode of operation.

Having accumulated power – and gained the blessing of Church and State – Savile used this power to abuse. We can see in the Smith report that there were specific dynamics around each programme: here we utilise the example of *Top of the Pops*.

Young people would gather outside *Top of the Pops* broadcasts in order to meet both DJs and pop stars. It is clear that some 'fans' would welcome a sexual encounter – this is where the crucial issue arises around age and consent. A 19-year-old entering a consensual sexual encounter with a celebrity may be a regrettable element of modern culture, but it is neither abusive nor unlawful. The focus here is on sexual encounters with children and young people. Of the crimes outlined in the Smith report, 34 out of 76 of Savile's BBC victims were under 16; consent with under 16s is not an issue, as legally they are unable to consent. However, in Savile's case, consent was not sought in any case – his attacks were sudden, brutal and without preliminaries. The nature of these attacks is consistent with what Finkelhor and Browne call:

> *Traumatic sexualization* [which] refers to a process in which a child's sexuality (including both sexual feelings and sexual attitudes) is shaped in a developmentally inappropriate and interpersonally dysfunctional fashion as a result of sexual abuse. (Finkelhor and Browne, 1985: 2)

Celebrity for Savile worked as follows: celebrity provided the power to enable access (to events and premises), in Savile's abusive mind this gave him non-consensual access to people's bodies and it provided protection from exposure. Savile stated to many of his victims that no one would believe them because he was 'King Jimmy' (Smith, 2016a: 350) and therefore untouchable. It is interesting to note that Stuart Hall was referred to as the 'King of the BBC Manchester' (Smith, 2016b: 168).

The silence of the victims

Perhaps the most shocking aspect of Savile's abuse was that his victims were silenced by the fear of power and celebrity. Silence is a recurring theme of the Smith report (2016a: 286, for example). Whilst the method adopted by the inquiry is not explicit in the way the data is reported, it seems clear that the victims were asked: What happened? How did it make you feel? What did you do as a result? The overwhelming answer to what did you do as a result was that no third party was informed. Savile often intimidated his victims – he was after all 'King Jimmy' – into silence. In some cases, the Savile victims told either BBC staff or family members, but it is disturbing that when victims did tell they were often told something along the lines 'that is just Jimmy' by BBC staff (Smith, 2016a: 409), again providing a parallel with Stuart Hall (Smith, 2016b: 136): it was seen as pointless challenging someone of Savile's celebrity standing. It should be recalled that as well as the high-profile celebrity standing Savile also had accumulated celebrity advantage through his Papal award, knighthood and charity fundraising efforts. This gave Savile what we have conceptualised as 'accumulated celebrity power', which in turn strengthened his ability to silence victims. This utilisation of power in turn generates relative power-lessness amongst his victims, a phenomenon noted by Finkelhor and Browne as follows:

> *Powerlessness* – or what might also be called disempowerment, the dynamic of rendering the victim powerless – refers to the process in which the child's will, desires, and sense of efficacy are continually contravened. Many aspects of the sexual abuse experience contribute to this dynamic. We theorize that a basic kind of powerlessness occurs in sexual abuse when a child's territory and body space are repeatedly invaded against the child's will. (Finkelhor and Browne, 1985: 3)

It is this sense of powerlessness that in turn generates the silence of the victims. The scale of Savile's abuse – not only at the BBC but in many other settings – makes the overwhelming silence even more remarkable.

The institutionalised nature of the abuse

This case study has explored Savile's abusive acts in the particular context of the BBC. However, the reader should note that he also abused in other institutional-ised settings: schools and hospitals in particular. It is argued here that the BBC in many ways facilitated Savile's abusive practices. The Smith report outlines some of these: for example, the notional age to take part in the *Top of the Pops* audience was 16, but this was poorly administered so that younger people were allowed in. Many witnesses to the Smith inquiry were aware that many young people in the audience were under 16 – indeed in one tragic case a young woman took her own life at the age of 15, when she was already an established *Top of the Pops* audience member and dancer (Smith, 2016a: 81). Clearly this was just one example of a policy inadequately implemented by the BBC. The Smith report also identifies three 'wake up calls' (2016a: 8) missed by the BBC, any one of which could have raised awareness of Savile's behaviour years or even decades before if it had come to light.

The *Top of the Pops* 'gaze' is relevant here to our discussion of institutional context and culture. The stage was set with DJs presenting whilst surrounded by adoring, mainly female fans (Smith, 2016a: 506). Savile took advantage of this by abusing young women in close proximity whilst on camera. One young woman can be seen jumping in shock when Savile's right hand is touching her intimately below the camera line. The cultural environment adds to the stigma felt by the victims, which many survivor statements to the Smith inquiry outline. This is theorised by Finkelhor and Browne as follows:

Stigmatization occurs in various degrees in different abusive situations. Some children are treated as bad and blameworthy by offenders and some are not. Some children, in the wake of a sexual abuse experience, are told clearly that they are not at fault, whereas others are heavily shamed. Some children may be too young to have much awareness of social attitudes and thus experience little stigmatization, whereas others have to deal with powerful religious and cultural taboos in addition to the usual stigma. (Finkelhor and Browne, 1985: 4)

The *Top of the Pops* camera also chooses to 'gaze' at attractive, young, usually female dancers – it is alleged in the Smith report that the audience were selected using 'attractiveness' as a criterion for entrance. Unfortunately, the report author falls into the trap of the 'attractiveness' criterion by evaluating some witnesses using this measure (Smith, 2016a: 383). If 'celebrity' is the problem then the BBC are clearly culpable in promoting a culture around 'celebrity' and 'talent' (the word used to describe presenters) in the organisation. The reader should note that it is probably the case that the celebrity culture has expanded since the Savile era: witness for example *Celebrity Big Brother, Strictly Come Dancing* and the wide range of other 'celebrity-based' programming. There is therefore no room for complacency: if celebrity offers a power base for abuse then the twenty-first century is probably more dangerous that the twentieth century ever was. Safeguarding practitioners should be aware of this possibility.

Reflection point

Thinking about celebrity abuse, is it possible that such extensive abuse could exist today?

Explore the Twitter feed for the #MeToo campaign.

What can be done to prevent such abuse by powerful, celebrity men?

By exploring the case of Jimmy Savile we have been able to gain valuable insights into celebrity abuse but also into the wider dynamics of child abuse such as the silencing of victims and how institutions collude with this. We explore institutional forms of abuse more extensively in Case Study Two, below, thus making a link between the two case studies.

Case study two: Abuse in institutional settings

It has emerged in recent decades that thousands of children have been abused in a whole range of institutions – schools, children's homes, sporting clubs and churches amongst them – throughout the twentieth century (McNeish and Scott, 2018). This form of abuse shares the features of all child abuse, that it is fundamentally the abuse of power over children and young people. In addition it has the particular feature of being located in institutions – settings with formal rules, regulations and official forms of authority. The extent of this abuse is really quite remarkable. Although there seem to be no comprehensive global studies of incidence, the cases involving the Roman Catholic Church cover many countries, including the United States of America, Spain, Italy, the United Kingdom and Australia (Astbury, 2013; Gallagher, 2000). The extent and geographical spread strongly suggests that this phenomenon cannot be explained by an individualist model (the one 'bad apple' or the lone pae-dophile) and that a more developed, theoretically based approach is required. This section attempts to work towards such a theory.

Towards a theory of institutional abuse

Looking back to the twentieth century it is apparent that child abuse existed across many forms of formal organisation and institutions (Gallagher, 2000). Before this the data is more difficult to gather but it would be surprising if this was not the case in boarding schools and church-based organisations, throughout the 1800s, for example. It may also be the case that forms of abuse exist in contemporary institu-tions: although it is noteworthy that fewer large institutions for children exist today largely due to the anti-institutional turn following allegations of abuse.

Any explanatory framework for understanding the extent of institutional abuse rests on the deployment of power in institutions. The classic sociological account of this can be found in Erving Goffman's *Asylums* (1961). Goffman developed the term 'total institution' to describe sites where all human life takes place in one institution – work, eating, leisure, social relations are all situated in one location. He describes in detail life in a mental hospital, an analysis which can be applied to other total institutions, including prisons or the armed forces. For Goffman these institutions are 'forcing houses for changing persons: each is a natural experiment on what can be done to the self' (1961: 22). His analysis can be applied to institu-tions which are more relevant to this book, even though they are not total institutions as such, including church-based organisations (Astbury, 2013), children's homes (Frost et al., 1999) and children's sports clubs (Hartill, 2014). In *Asylums* Goffman describes how inmates are stripped of identity, subject to imposed regimes and routines and obliged to accept forms of control and authority. The danger of these situations can be seen in relation to abuse: power is located in particular individuals and forms of authority, the inmates are subordinated to this authority through the deployment of power and the institutional practices are more or less closed off from the outside world.

We can see this – perhaps in its most globally extensive form – in the Roman Catholic Church: here we see a link with the Savile case study that we have already discussed. In the church, authority rests with the official representative – the priest or bishop, for example. It is very difficult to challenge this as the authority is granted through the power of God. The victim, again as in the Savile case, feels unable to speak out as they fear that they will not be believed when they are speaking out against a person with considerable status and authority. This is remarkably an oft repeated story by children who have been abused in church settings, children's homes and by football coaches alike: they report that they feel that no one will believe them, and indeed they are often told this by the abuser (Brackenridge, 2001; Smith, 2016a). Abuse is usually followed by silence and then by disbelief. The silence is individualised at first but when the institution is challenged the disbelief and silencing are often institutionalised – again the early, and sometimes ongoing, denial by the Roman Catholic Church provides an example of this.

Thus, a theory can be constructed as follows: institutions are sites where power is embedded in practices and in designated individuals. Where these individuals decide to breach established social norms through sexual abuse the victim usually feels unable to speak out due to the power and status of the abuser: often the entire institution (church, children's home or school) can continue the silence and denial (Lovett et al., 2018).

Forms of abuse

When one reads the now numerous reports on institutional abuse the pattern is alarmingly similar. Initially the institutions are held in high regard – they can be faith-based, run by the State or respected elements of the voluntary sector or high-prestige sports or cultural institutions. It is difficult to assess if perpetrators are attracted to such establishments or if the abuse is more opportunistic and situational – examples of both seem to exist. As we saw in the analysis of the Jimmy Savile case previously, grooming takes place as a key mechanism leading to abuse. Institutions form a base where grooming can take place: there may be locations for the abuse to occur, the perpetrator may be able to use awards (trips out, sweets, extra privileges) to make the child feel special and separate them out from their peer group (Barter, 1999). The child will often be dependent on the adult for many of their emotional and practical needs. The grooming process will often extend to family networks – with promises of places in sports teams, for example, being highlighted as part of this process. Families may well look up to the perpetrator and regard them as having a special role in looking after the needs of their child. As with all forms of sexual abuse the perpetrators are likely to be male, but unlike most other forms of abuse the victims too are often male, unlike the statistics outlined in Table 3.1, for example (McNeish and Scott, 2018). The exact nature of the abuse varies from case to case but often involves forms of penetrative sex and oral sex. From the many disturbing incidents outlined in the now numerous inquiries we select just one to illustrate the point. The outline is graphic and explicit:

> It is difficult to describe the appalling sexual abuse inflicted over decades on children aged as young as seven at Ampleforth School, and 11 at Downside School. Ten individuals, mostly monks, connected to these two institutions have been convicted or cautioned in relation to offences involving sexual activity with a large number of children, or offences concerning pornography. The true scale of the abuse however is likely to be considerably higher. Some examples of the abuse are set out below. Piers Grant-Ferris was convicted of 20 counts of indecent assault against 15 boys who attended the junior school at Ampleforth. A victim of Piers Grant-Ferris described how he had made him remove his clothes in the confessional of the chapel, then beat his bare bottom. Another incident took place in a bathroom when he was forced to strip naked and to place his hands and feet on each side of a bathtub, so he was straddling the bath, with his genitals hanging down. He was then beaten on his bare bottom, an event he found 'absolutely terrifying'. During these repeated beatings, Grant-Ferris would masturbate. (IICSA, 2018: iii)

People often ask why children do not tell someone after one incident of abuse has occurred and why children find themselves in situations where they may be re-abused. Whilst this process is at first puzzling it can be understood using our theoretical framework developed in the Savile case study discussed earlier. Re-abuse occurs because:

1 Abusers carry considerable power which makes victims reluctant to speak out
2 Children and young people understand that they may well be disbelieved when the abuser carries the authority of, say, a priest, a football coach or a residential care worker
3 The children and young people may have been threatened with retaliation if they tell anyone about the abuse – for example, a loss of privileges in care settings or not being selected for a sports team.

It is not surprising then that abuse in institutional settings is often sustained, repetitive and serious.

Building safe organisations and institutions

It is clear that organised settings – ranging from total institutions (such as youth custody settings) to day care settings for under-fives – can be dangerous places for children, where they can be vulnerable to sexual and other forms of abuse. The implications for challenging these forms of abuse are discussed below.

Reducing the numbers of institutionalised children

Increasing awareness of sexual abuse, a shift away from authoritarian settings, a belief in family-based care, the impact of academic literature (Goffman, 1961) and of popular cultural artefacts (films such as *One Flew Over the Cuckoo's Nest, Rabbit Proof Fence* and *The Magdalene Sisters*) have all contributed to a decline in both the number of and the size of welfare institutions. However, we should not be complacent: globally it is estimated that 8 million children live in orphanages and other institutions (www.wearelumos.org). In the British child welfare sector, however, there are now very few large residential settings for children in the public sector, whereas from the 1970s onwards large homes known as Community Homes (Education) were predominant. Of the 75,420 children in care in England in 2018, 9,990 were in some form of residential care, most of these being small settings. We note with some irony that such settings still exist in the fee-paying, private education setting and have sometimes been identified as not always safe (as illustrated by the quote in our earlier section from Ampleforth, IICSA, 2018).

Making existing institutions safer

It is not possible – and some would argue it is undesirable – to end all institutionalised care for children. If we widen the debate it is also important for children to engage in sports and cultural activities which involve some kind of organisation and structure, usually in the care of adults. In many ways Goffman's work on the total institutions can be used in reverse to indicate what good care looks like. Goffman wrote of the stripping of identity, the imposition of routines and depersonalisation – all practices which should be avoided in truly caring environments (Erooga, 2009). Institutions can be made safe environments by:

1   Employing safe recruitment practices. This has been the most widely implemented reform in residential and day care for example. In England services exist such as the Disclosure and Barring Service (DBS) which screen applicants for posts to ensure they do not have a known criminal record. Whilst this is a useful

safeguarding service it should be noted that many perpetrators, particularly of sexual abuse, are not known to the criminal justice system.

2   Peter Drucker, the eminent leadership scholar, is often quoted as stating that 'culture eats strategy for breakfast' (Whitzman, 2016). This is relevant in this debate as it is the culture and the values of the staff and the organisation that really matter. A staff member who is truly child-centred will be safe in the company of children. The organisation will be protective and will organise any child-centred activity around a strong value base, with an inclusive leadership model, which models the application of appropriate values.

3   Taking Goffman's work (1961) as suggesting what is oppressive and potentially abusive it follows that the more open and porous an organisation is the better it will be at safeguarding children. Depending on the exact nature of the organisation, practices such as lay visiting, peer review, fully engaged management committees and open days will all contribute to a transparent culture which is less likely to be abusive.

4   Genuine participation by children and young people will encourage respect for them as people in their own right and not as 'objects of concern' to use the words of Butler-Sloss in her report on the situation in Cleveland (1988).

Reflection point

Having read the section above about institutional care and abuse:

Think about an organisation or institution you know: is it safe for children and what could be done to make it safer?

Conclusion

The aims of this chapter have been to:

- Explore the phenomenon of abuse by celebrities: developing the concept of 'accumulated celebrity abuse'
- Explore abuse of children and young people in institutional settings
- Apply learning from these settings to our theoretical and practical understanding of child abuse.

Whilst this chapter has focused on two specific case studies – abuse by celebrities and abuse in institutional settings – much of the learning is transferable. The chapter has illustrated the nature of abuse outside of the household. The abuse of power and the silencing of victims are features of both these case studies and can be seen in cases of abuse within the family and in contextual exploitation situations as well. Given the high profile of such abuse cases one would hope that in the contemporary environment such widespread abuse cannot exist – but it would be naive to think like this, as abuse is hidden and secretive as we have seen.

Recommended reading

Di McNeish and Sara Scott, *Key Messages from Research on Institutional Child Sexual Abuse* (2018)

This report summarises the key findings on child sexual abuse in institutional settings in an accessible and easy to read format.

Dame Janet Smith, *The Jimmy Savile Investigation Report* (2016)

This report explains how widespread institutional abuse can occur and explores the practices that enabled this. Savile is probably the most prolific sex offender in British history and the narrative will resonate with those who came across his work during their childhood. Savile's mode of operation is shared in other celebrity scandals, and resembles in many ways some of the issues uncovered by the #MeToo movement.

5

ASSESSING NEED AND PROVIDING EARLY HELP

CONTENTS

The aims of this chapter are to:

- Understand the importance of family support and offering 'early help'
- Reflect on the role of assessment in safeguarding children and young people
- Consider the skills required in assessment and support practice
- Analyse the role of multi-professional working in assessment and support practice

Introduction

Assessment is an essential safeguarding skill which will be explored in this chapter. As part of this exploration, early help, or family support, which underpins safeguarding, but is too often underplayed and under-funded, will be outlined and analysed. The case will be made for the central role of family support in both preventing child abuse and promoting social justice. The key role of universal services (schools and health) will be emphasised in terms of their fundamental role in the provision of services in supporting children and young people and their families. The focus here is on the assessment of 'children in need' (under Section 17 of the Children Act 1989) although assessments may take place for other purposes: early years and special education needs, for example.

Providing family support

'Family support' is a term that can be used to define professional and community-based practices which are sometimes identified as prevention, early intervention or early help (for a full discussion of mobilisation of these terms see Frost et al., 2015). The basic argument here is that family support can be offered by practitioners and third sector agencies to support families and prevent the emergence or worsening of safeguarding issues. The term 'early help' is utilised in *Working Together to Safeguard Children* (HMG, 2018), which in turn draws on the review undertaken by Professor Eileen Munro (2011) on behalf of the then UK Coalition government. It is argued in this book that there are shortcomings implicit in the use of the early help concept – 'early' is suggestive of predictive powers which do not really exist and being in receipt of 'help' suggests that the recipients are passive, rather than active participants.

Reflection point

The provision of services to families to stop any problems getting worse can be referred to as prevention OR early help OR early intervention OR family support.

Which term is most widely used in your workplace / course?

Do you have a term that you personally prefer?

If so, why is this?

Family support is underpinned by statute: there is legal support in England in Section 17 of the Children Act 1989, and across the nations of the United Kingdom (Northern Ireland, Scotland and Wales) there are different formulations in providing legal support for family support service provision. The legal mandate is important here in demonstrating that the provision of such support services is indeed part of a statute – practitioners often make the mistake of referring to safeguarding work as somehow 'statutory' and family support as not falling into this category. This is a serious error with potentially profound policy and political effects: to reiterate, family support and early help are provided under a statute and are an essential element of safeguarding. There is also notably an international mandate in the United Nations Convention on the Rights of the Child – see Article 19.1 of the Convention reproduced in the box below.

Article 19 United Nations Convention on the Rights of the Child

1   States Parties shall take all appropriate legislative, administrative, social and educational measures to protect the child from all forms of physical or mental violence, injury or abuse, neglect or negligent treatment, maltreatment or exploitation, including sexual abuse, while in the care of parent(s), legal guardian(s) or any other person who has the care of the child.
2   Such protective measures should, as appropriate, include effective procedures for the establishment of social programmes to provide necessary support for the child and for those who have the care of the child, as well as for other forms of prevention and for identification, reporting, referral, investigation, treatment and follow-up of instances of child maltreatment described heretofore, and, as appropriate, for judicial involvement.

Mary Daly and colleagues have produced a global overview of family and parenting support where they argue that:

> Family support varies widely in practice ... services tend to be problem-oriented rather than preventive, although there are increasing moves towards a preventive orientation. (Daly et al., 2015: 15)

It is argued here that the safeguarding of children and young people should be underpinned by the practice of family support and further that high quality safeguarding practices should operate alongside family support practices. There is a danger that without an emphasis on family support, safeguarding becomes authoritarian in nature and as a result safeguarding will exacerbate the impact of social divisions meaning that interventions tend to focus on poorer families disproportionately. This argument has powerfully been made by, amongst others, four influential British-based professors – Brid Featherstone, Anna Gupta, Kate Morris and Sue White (Featherstone et al., 2014, 2018). Whilst this book takes a position similar to these two publications it also differs: here we take multi-disciplinary approach whereas Featherstone and colleagues focus on social work, which, it can be argued, leads to some misplaced judgements in their publications. They also imply that a child-focused approach is somehow unethical, which is a position that the author of this book would distance himself from.

It is also important to note here that family support is fully consistent with the public service professional values that will be shared by many readers of this book. Family support is based in what we can identify as partnership working, empowering practice, strengths-based and relationship-based and restorative practices, forms of practice which all practitioners can support. Family support is a practice that has a powerful and social impact in improving the lives of children, young people and their families.

Reflection point

In your professional role, or the one you are training or volunteering for, what emphasis is placed on family support compared to the emphasis placed on safeguarding?

Is one focus emphasised rather than the other?

How do you feel about this in relation to your values?

In this book it is argued that family support should be centre stage and that safeguarding practice should be based in family support values and approaches.

Adverse childhood experiences

The concept of adverse childhood experiences (ACEs) provides a lens for exploring and understanding assessment and family support issues. In the field of child welfare and safeguarding there are often new trends and different ways of perceiving the issues that emerge – and very often these trends fade and new directions emerge.

In recent years there has been a focus on negative childhood experiences – identified as ACEs – which have been identified as being linked with disadvantages faced later in adult life. The leading international scholar on the field of child protection – David Finkelhor – writes on this subject as follows:

> The Adverse Childhood Experiences research has quickly grown into the lodestar in the United States for much policy discussion in the child maltreatment field. (Finkelhor, 2018: 174)

This section of the book provides an analysis and balanced critique of the ACEs approach.

What are ACEs?

Adverse childhood experiences have become a lens through which we can understand negative childhood experiences and their perceived link to adult outcomes. The policy aim of this particular approach is to challenge, and thereby reduce, childhood ACEs and then as a consequence to improve adult lives and enhance positive outcomes. The United States-based scholars Felitti et al. (1998) are credited with the conception and early work in relation to ACEs – a recurrent theme as we have seen earlier in this book is that the USA can have a powerful influence on UK perspectives and across the English-speaking world. In 1998 Felitti and colleagues published the results of a survey of adults to assess whether they had experienced ACEs. Seven types of ACEs were surveyed: psychological, physical and sexual abuse; violence against the mother; or living with household members who were substance abusers, mentally ill or suicidal; and whether the participant had ever been imprisoned. Felitti et al. report that 9,508 people responded to the survey – a return rate of 70.5 per cent. The research team explain their analysis of the findings as follows:

> Logistic regression was used to adjust for effects of demographic factors on the association between the cumulative number of categories of childhood exposures (range: 0–7) and risk factors for the leading causes of death in adult life. (Felitti et al., 1998: 245)

Their analysis found that around half the respondents had experienced one or more ACEs and that about one-quarter of respondents had experienced two or more. Where people had experienced four or more ACEs (what the researchers call the 'dose') there was up to a 12-fold increase in serious health problems in adulthood. The American research team therefore conclude as follows:

> We found a strong graded relationship between the breadth of exposure to abuse or household dysfunction during childhood and multiple risk factors for several of the leading causes of death in adults. (Felitti et al., 1998: 245)

As Finkelhor (2018) points out, the average age of the respondents to the original Felitti survey was 55 years, the childhood experiences were a considerable time ago, and that current issues may be different. However, the findings remain striking and help to explain why ACEs have indeed become a 'lodestar' (the guiding light), to use Finkelhor's term.

We should, however, be wary of the uncritical transfer of research findings from the United States where specific social factors (such as the lack of a welfare infrastructure and a strong association between poverty and particular ethnicities) may mean that findings do not transfer elsewhere in a straightforward manner. There are, helpfully, more recent and more geographically relevant surveys in the UK setting, an oft-quoted one being that undertaken in Wales during 2015. The findings are summarised as follows:

> For every 100 adults in Wales, 47 had at least one ACE during their childhood and 14 experienced four or more. After correcting for socio-demographics, ACE counts predicted health-harming behaviours (four or more ACEs vs none) – e.g. violence victimisation (adjusted odds ratio 14·2, 95% CI 9·1–22·1; p<0·0001), high-risk drinking (4·4, 3·1–6·4; p<0·0001), and low mental well-being (4·7, 3·4–6·4; p<0·0001). Furthermore, modelling suggested that health-harming behaviours and low mental well-being nationally could be attributed to ACEs. (Ashton et al., 2016: 21)

The actual impact on adult experiences suggested by the Welsh survey is outlined in the box below.

. . . .

Impact of ACEs – Welsh government survey

4× more likely to be a high-risk drinker

16× more likely to have used crack cocaine or heroin

6× increased risk of never or rarely feeling optimistic

3× increased risk of heart disease, respiratory disease and type 2 diabetes

15× more likely to have committed violence

14× more likely to have been a victim of violence in the last 12 months

20× more likely to have been in prison at any point in their life

. . . .

These findings are consistent with those undertaken in the USA and we can argue, with some confidence, that there is indeed a strong association between ACEs and poor outcomes in adulthood. As Finkelhor (2018) points out, in this case we need to consider what is the mediating factor – addressing the question of exactly how does an ACE result in a poor adult outcome? What is the mechanism that leads to any link? The literature tends to focus on either neurobiological or psycho-social factors as the key mediating factors: that is, changes in the brain or body as a result of ACEs or changes in social functioning and well-being.

Challenges to the ACEs perspective

An important element of being an effective safeguarding professional is being able to think critically and reflect on approaches and data. Whilst the ACEs approach is in many ways helpful, it can be argued that there are a number of problems inherent in the approach: these are outlined and discussed below.

An over-individualised approach

One issue for the ACEs approach is that it is in danger of presenting an over-individualised approach – it implies that the core of child abuse rests in individual experiences in individualised households. This rests uneasily with more social structural approaches, which, for example, would place more emphasis on class, poverty and inequality. In relation to social class there is certainly a strong association between being drawn to the attention of Children's Social Care services and living in poverty. Many research studies, for example those led by Paul Bywaters (Bywaters et al., 2016a, 2016b) in the UK, have pointed to the association between living in poverty and being identified as a child in need or a child requiring child protection services. Some ACE-based approaches accommodate poverty and social class, but some do not. In response to some ACEs work, again undertaken in Wales, Taylor-Robinson and colleagues (2018) make a powerful case for a social structural approach and the provision of universal services to tackle ACEs, thus moving away from the individualised approach:

> Our contention is that efforts to improve child health outcomes should focus on reducing modifiable socio-economic inequalities, as well as early identification and appropriate intervention for children that have had adverse childhood experiences, which will vary widely depending on the specific exposure. The concept of adverse childhood experiences has been a useful starting point for debates about investing in children's health, but it should not obscure the overarching idea of important, modifiable, determinants of child health. (Taylor-Robinson et al., 2018: 263)

Underplaying resilience

There is a body of research which has a focus on resilience in childhood: resilience is usually seen as being able to respond to and overcome adversity (Gilligan, 2000). We have all faced challenges in our lives and we can reflect how resilient, or not, we were in the face of these adversities. Practitioners can work with children and young people to build their resilience and help them confront problems, as Gilligan (2000) points out. Resilience seems to come primarily from positive relationships and a resultant sense of self-esteem. This is one reason why people who have experienced sexual abuse often identify themselves as 'survivors' rather than 'victims' – thus demonstrating their resilience. The ACEs approach is in danger of being over-deterministic, meaning that it can imply that a negative childhood experience inevitably leads to poor adult outcomes, thus underplaying the role of resilience.

Predicting outcomes: False positives and false negatives

The ability of practitioners and researchers to make predictions is often over-rated in the child protection field. In this context this means that some people with ACEs will not experience adult adversity, and some people who have not experienced ACEs may face problems in adulthood. These are known in the literature as 'false positives' or 'false negatives' (Munro, 1999). Finkelhor (2018), in his critical analysis of the ACEs approach, argues that this prediction issue is a problem and quotes a dementia study where for every four cases that were positively identified there were 23 false cases identified.

Focus on problems not strengths

Perhaps most problematically for the ACEs approach, in recent years practitioners have tended to focus on the positives of even the most challenging situations: this is often identified as strengths-based practice or restorative practice and is reflected in techniques such as Signs of Safety or in Family Group Conferences (Frost and Jackson, 2018).

Bronfenbrenner's work can be utilised to warn against the potentially over-determinist and negative focus of the ACEs approach. He argues, for example, that a single positive relationship can help children overcome adversity:

> Proposition 1: In order to develop intellectually, emotionally, socially and morally a child requires participation in progressively more complex reciprocal activity on a regular basis over an extended period in the child's life, with one or more persons with whom the child develops a strong, mutual, irrational, emotional attachment and who is committed to the child's well-being and development, preferably for life. (Bronfenbrenner, 1991: 2)

Bronfenbrenner translated this principle effectively into simple and very powerful terms as follows:

> Every child needs at least one adult who is irrationally crazy about him or her. (Bronfenbrenner, 1991: 2)

This optimistic approach by Bronfenbrenner helps to illustrate how people can positively survive even the most negative childhood experiences if the necessary care, love and support are in place.

Reflection point

How useful do you find an approach to safeguarding embedded in an adverse childhood experiences perspective?

What are the strengths and weaknesses of the ACEs approach?

Safeguarding children and social inequalities

As we have seen in the discussion above, the issue of ACEs is closely related to the debates about the impact of poverty and inequality on child welfare in general, and, in this context, on safeguarding in particular. There is a long history of association between child welfare work and poverty – it is, however, a history that it is often invisible in discussions of safeguarding (Featherstone et al., 2014). In recent years, in the United Kingdom context, the work of Paul Bywaters and colleagues has been invaluable in shedding light on inequality and the relationship to safeguarding. Some of their key findings are outlined in the box below.

Bywaters et al. (2016b): summary of key findings

- Each improvement in socio-economic circumstances leads to a lower proportion of children looked after (CLA) and on child protection plans (CPP)
- Children in the poorest 10 per cent of local areas are 10 times more likely to be CLA or on a CPP
- [There is a] Strong relationship between being in poverty and being in receipt of CSC (Children's Social Care) services
- Impact of ethnicity is complex – with Black Caribbean children more likely to be CLA than White children
- Poor/missing data on poverty/disability
- Variations between different local authorities with similar deprivation rates

There is, as the evidence here indicates, a powerful connection between poverty and professional safeguarding responses: this helps to highlight the importance of family support services, which recognise the impact of poverty.

Providing family support

Children and young people will often come to the attention of practitioners as potentially being 'children in need': frequently these children and young people will be living in poverty. A social worker may be dealing with a referral about a child who in a day care setting seems neglected, a health visitor may be concerned about the standard of parental care, a teacher may be worried about a child who always seems to be hungry or a police officer may deal with a 'home alone' child. They all need to work together if they are to deliver effective family support. The English Children Act 1989, for example, defines a 'child in need' in the following circumstances:

1   he is unlikely to achieve or maintain, or to have the opportunity of achieving or maintaining, a reasonable standard of health or development without the provision for him of services by a local authority under this Part;
2   his health or development is likely to be significantly impaired, or further impaired, without the provision for him of such services; or
3   he is disabled.

The Act refers to 'family' as including 'any person who has parental responsibility for the child and any other person with whom he has been living'. The reference to 'he' is in the original Act and legally refers to all children and young people under the age of 18.

The Children Act 1989, also establishes a 'general duty' therefore for local authorities to safeguard and promote the welfare of children and families who are in need, as follows:

1   It shall be the general duty of every local authority (in addition to the other duties imposed on them by this Part)—

    a   to safeguard and promote the welfare of children within their area who are in need; and
    b   so far as is consistent with that duty, to promote the upbringing of such children by their families,

by providing a range and level of services appropriate to those children's needs.

Effective family support services should be designed to reflect this concept by ensuring that there is a range of community family support services in each local area so that 'early help' can prevent the escalation of family challenges.

Conceptual issues

Family support can be utilised to address the range of ACEs, for example, addressing neglect, forms of trauma and issues such as bullying, or working with substance misuse or mental health problems of parents or carers. There is a degree of international recognition for the utilisation of the term family support (Canavan et al., 2006; Daly et al., 2015). Family support is consistent with the United Nations Convention on the Rights of the Child (UNCRC) which has influenced the international range of Children Acts which followed the UNCRC. Family support is traditionally perceived as difficult to conceptualise and to define – it has been referred to as a 'slippery concept' (Frost et al., 2015: 3). This may be because family support consists of a range of practices, and draws on a wide range of theories including sociology, psychology and social policy: it is thus harder to define as an activity than say 'teaching' or 'policing'. Perhaps this diversity and complexity is one reason that family support has been difficult to defend in times of austerity experienced since the global financial crisis of 2008.

It is argued here that family support has the following identifying characteristics:

1   Family support offers inclusive and engaging practices based on the idea of offering support to families, children and young people who feel they require such support. Family support is therefore strongly suggestive of partnership, engagement and consent.
2   Such support can be offered early in the life of the child or early in the emergence of the identified challenge facing the family: this is why it is sometimes referred to as 'early help'. It is important that family support services can be relevant to all children and young people, and not only to younger children.
3   Family support is a pro-active process which engages with the parent(s) and/ or child or young person in a positive process of change. Implicit in the term family support is the suggestion of bringing about change within the family and social network and being based in a theory of change.
4   Family support attempts to prevent the emergence, or worsening, of family challenges, or ACEs if we wish to use that particular terminology.
5   Family support also aims to generate wider social change and benefits. Such results may lead to a saving in public expenditure, a decrease in social problems, an improvement in the quality of family life or a reduction in measurable outcomes, such as the number of children coming into care.

Thinking about family support has often utilised what is known as the Hardiker model (Hardiker et al., 1991) which sees family support as existing at three levels:

- Primary prevention refers to universal programmes, often area-based and embedded in families and communities. Where practitioners are involved they work on an agreed basis with a wide range of families. There should be no stigma attached to using such services as the aim can be seen as preventing the emergence of family problems. Examples of primary prevention projects may include summer play schemes, adventure playgrounds, toy libraries and children's centres.

- Secondary prevention is aimed at families with an identified challenge, who usually recognise these issues themselves and who wish to work with agencies towards change through a support and partnership model. Challenges may include parenting, isolation and low-level mental health challenges, for example. Secondary prevention may include volunteer home visiting programmes, such as Home Start, or service provision by family support workers, based in the statutory sector or the third sector (Frost et al., 2000).

- Tertiary prevention is conceptualised as being at the 'heavier' or perhaps more 'targeted' end of a family support spectrum. It may focus on issues such as drug or alcohol misuse, domestic abuse or mental ill-health. Tertiary prevention may also involve working with children on the 'edge of care'. This may be delivered by a range of practitioners – probably working in more specialised fields than those working at secondary prevention.

This classification of levels is helpful as it can be utilised to assess the availability and delivery of services at each level in a given geographical area.

Reflection point

The terms 'early help', 'prevention', 'family support' and 'early intervention' have meanings that overlap but give different focus to policy and practice.

Do you have a preference? If so why is this your preference? Are you aware of any significant geographical differences?

What is the evidence for family support?

Perhaps the highest profile example of positive evidence in relation to family support comes from the United States project known as the *HighScope Perry Pre-school Program* (Schweinhart et al., 2005). The programme operated in an inner city area of Michigan during the 1960s, and was designed as a family support and educational programme that worked with African-American children aged between three and five years of age. The programme consisted of two and a half hours per day of centre-based day care for the children during the week which operated alongside a series of home visits. Whilst the actual project is similar to many across the world, it is particularly significant as it utilised extensive research which followed up the children at 15, 19, 27 and 40 years of age. The children involved in the study were allocated to an intervention group and a control group: 58 children in the intervention group and 65 in the control group, the latter did not receive the service. The attrition rate during the research period was low for such a long-term project and the researchers were still in contact with approximately 90 per cent of the group at the time of the fortieth birthday follow-up.

The outcomes of the programme are complex and sometimes contested, but can be summarised as in the box below.

Summary of Perry HighScope findings (Schweinhart et al., 2005: 2)

The programme children:

Are less likely to be arrested 5 times or more (36% as opposed to 55% of the control group)

Are more likely to earn $20k plus (60% as opposed to 40%)

Are more likely to graduate from high school (77% as opposed to 60%)

Achieve more highly at 15 (49% as opposed to 15%)

Are more likely to complete homework (61% as opposed to 38%)

Are more likely to have an IQ of 90+ at 5 (67% as opposed to 28%)

In the light of these findings the researchers concluded that:

High quality pre-school programs for young children living in poverty contribute to their intellectual and social development in childhood and their school success, economic performance, and reduced commission of crime in adulthood. This study confirms that these findings extend not only to young adults, but also to adults in midlife. It confirms that the long-term effects are lifetime effects. The Perry Pre-school study indicates that the return to the public on its initial investment in such programs is not only substantial but larger than previously estimated. (Schweinhart et al., 2005: 6)

Bellfield et al. undertook an overall cost–benefit analysis of Perry HighScope and concluded that $12.90 was saved from public expenditure for every $1 invested and therefore argue that 'program gains come mainly from reduced crime by males' (2006: 1).

The strongest comparable English evidence relevant to family support is probably that collected by the LARC (Local Authority Research Consortium) in their study of a shared assessment and intervention model known as the Common Assessment Framework (CAF): the study is known as LARC4. The LARC4 methodology can be outlined as follows:

> Eleven of the twelve LARC4 local authorities carried out their own qualitative case study research projects within an overall agreed framework developed by the LAs [local authorities] and NFER [National Foundation for Educational Research]. Each case study involved interviews with LA practitioners, parents and (where appropriate) children and young people. In all, the LAs conducted around 80 interviews across 39 case studies between spring and autumn 2011. Each case study looked at whether the common assessment process is a cost-effective way to support improved outcomes and avoid costly negative outcomes for families later on. (Easton et al., 2012: Foreword)

The LARC4 study also explored how to assess the costs and/or savings of implementing the family support, a notoriously difficult issue to measure:

> To calculate a difference in costs (i.e. an indicative 'saving'), LARC adopted the adapted 'futures methodology' … Futures methodologies are increasingly being used within research and evaluation to ascertain what might have happened if, for example, an intervention had not been implemented. LARC4 LAs asked practitioners, parents and, where appropriate, children/young people for their perceptions on what the life course of a child/family might have been had the CAF process not been initiated. LARC LA leads then moderated all the case studies. (Easton et al., 2012: Foreword)

The key findings of the LARC4 study are summarised in the report Foreword as follows:

- Outcomes for children, young people and their families experiencing problems can be improved – and in some cases very dramatically – by appropriate interventions planned and managed by services working effectively together
- The Common Assessment Framework (CAF) process encourages, and provides a good basis for, such integrated planning and intervention
- There are five key success factors for early intervention, all of which should be present

- The costs of working and intervening in this joined-up way are likely to be repaid many times over by the avoidance of greater costs later in the life of the child or family (although not all of the savings will accrue at the local service level).

Bullet point three above refers to 'five key success factors' which are as follows (Easton et al., 2012: 21), and give an important direction for practitioners:

- Engaging children, young people and families as equal partners in the process
- Ensuring consistency of the lead professional support, which helped families and practitioners work together better
- Integrating all of the elements of the CAF process, from holistic assessment, TAC (Team Around the Child) model and meetings, lead professional role, action planning and reviews
- Ensuring multi-agency working and information sharing, which improved understanding of need and service provision
- Developing a better understanding of children and young people's needs at the earliest possible stage.

The LARC4 research team summarised their findings as follows in helping us address the 'what works' question:

> A range of support interventions were put in place to help families. Most commonly help was given to enhance parenting strategies; improve engagement in education; develop emotional health and resilience; engage in positive activities and promote physical health management. Families reported that the informal help and support given by lead practitioners helped them manage their situations. (Easton et al., 2012: Summary)

The researchers estimated that the 'potential future outcome costs' of the cases they explored were between £400 and £420,000. The cost of undertaking the CAF and the intervention costs were between £1,500 and £27,000. It is argued therefore that 'potential savings' range from £6,800 and £415,000. This evidence suggests that this form of early intervention is cost-effective and, of course, a more humane process for the families concerned.

Reflection point

Do you find the evidence for family support convincing?

Do you know of the evidence that promotes any family support projects you work with or know of?

Supporting families

Universal services are fundamental to a caring and supportive society. Every family depends, to some degree, on universal support provided by practitioners such as midwives and health visitors, community-based services provided by playgroups, children's centres and schools: this is what Hardiker and her colleagues (1991) identify as primary prevention. These services are essential in supporting families and where they are well resourced and accessible they will reduce the incidence of child abuse and reduce child mortality rates. They reflect what is meant by the oft quoted African proverb that 'it takes a village to raise a child'.

Once these services have been accessed and if the needs increase it can necessitate a referral to children's social care services, triggering an assessment under the parameters of being a child in need. The child and family can experience a range of social care interventions, including home visiting (Howard and Brooks-Gunn, 2009), direct work and coordinated working with a range of agencies, all aimed at achieving change around the issue of the health, development and welfare of the child. This work could be about reducing any harmful effects of parental behaviours on the child's daily life, improving the home environment, improving health, education or well-being.

Frost et al. suggest that the essence of help at this stage is good quality support to families through 'partnership work that encourages and develops their resilience' (2015: 56). Effective, theoretically informed family support work draws on traditions of applying a strengths-based approach, which considers how life stressors can cause disruption to relationships, coping methods and support systems. There are several 'tools' that aid the practitioner to facilitate change and improved coping strategies such as genograms and eco-maps: these can be used in one-to-one, direct work sessions, with children, young people or adults.

As we have already argued, safeguarding practitioners have a duty to utilise research findings. There is, however, a challenge in researching family support, as research projects are attempting to research what has not happened: this is a complex research challenge. Godar argues that research in this field can play a fundamental role in service development involving the exploration of:

- Prevalence: how many children and families have a particular characteristic, or experience (e.g. number of children living with domestic violence)?
- Trends: is the number of children with a particular need changing over time? Are the types of needs that children experience changing?
- Relationships: is there a relationship between different characteristics and needs (e.g. the correlation between parental substance misuse and domestic violence)? Where a robust statistical analysis is carried out and shows a relationship between two factors, this is called correlation.

- Risk: does the presence of a particular need, or combination of needs, increase the probability of a later negative outcome (e.g. the increased risk that the children of young parents will not reach developmental milestones by the age of five)? (Godar 2013: 42)

Family support is essentially a humane and relationship-based process (Frost et al., 2015). Studies and programmes, particularly those in the United States and those supported by the Early Intervention Foundation, tend to focus on 'outcomes' which are the measurable results of family support rather than the nature of the support and the quality of the relationships which underpin this. The focus on the research method known as RCTs (randomised controlled trials) and the subsequent outcomes has undermined a focus on the 'process' of family support, which explores the means by which practitioners actually undertake their practice. What is required is research that takes a holistic approach taking into account the wider social context (Featherstone et al., 2014) and places due emphasis on both the 'process' of family support and the potential outcomes. This is required if we are to fully understand the complexities of family support and its crucial role in preventing child abuse. This is well stated by Pinkerton and Katz as follows:

> In any evaluation of family support, a balance must be struck between the demands of technically achievable, objective measures and the need to adequately represent and address the fundamental purpose of policy and practice. (2003: 16)

Canavan et al. make the case for reflective practice, informed by research, in relation to family support:

> Doing family support requires a mixture of description and questioning informed by action. It is a mixture which provides the basis for reflective practice. (2006: 17)

We return to the issue of reflection in Chapter 9 of this book.

Multi-professional assessment

Assessment is a key skill in delivering family support – certainly at the secondary and tertiary levels. In England over recent decades the assessment process has drawn on the assessment triangle which has proven to be remarkably robust and remains 'fit for purpose' during the 2020s, although the environmental aspects are arguably underplayed (Figure 5.1). The triangle includes the child's developmental needs, explores parenting capacity and examines the wider family and community context in which the child lives. The model draws on the work of the esteemed social scientist Urie Bronfenbrenner who perceived the child as living within a wider ecological system.

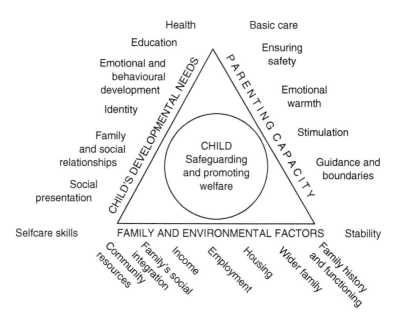

Figure 5.1   The assessment triangle – Working Together to Safeguard Children (HMG, 2018)

The originators of the assessment triangle should be praised for providing a robust tool that survived decades of social change and can still be used to assess the issue of 'contextual safeguarding', which is explored in Chapter 8.

There is an art to the assessment process – in this book we deliberately refer to an 'assessment process' as it should be undertaken as an active process, not as a static event undertaken by the professional with a passive, recipient family. In fact, any distinction between 'assessment' and 'intervention' is in many ways false: assessment is always an intervention as the professional presence will act as a change agent, and any intervention should also be constantly reassessed and reflected upon to take into account any changes and new information. A safeguarding assessment will be led by a qualified social worker, but all relevant practitioners should see themselves as part of this important process.

The purpose of assessment in the child and young person safeguarding context is:

1   to gather accurate information about the child or young person's life in the context of the household and the wider community

2   to provide an informed, evidence-based analysis of whether the child is at risk of 'serious harm'

3   to assess whether the child or young person can be offered family support in order to remain at home or if they require safeguarding by being placed outside of the home

4   to work together, wherever possible, with the child or young person, their families and carers to agree the strengths of the family and the nature of any challenges they face

5   to work together with the full range of relevant practitioners to gather useful and accurate information

6   to plan and where possible deliver services to ensure the child is safeguarded.

Your organisation will have protocols that will assist and guide practitioners in the assessment of children in need or children potentially in need of safeguarding, and if you are undertaking such an assessment you should use the support and supervision provided by your team and organisation. The assessment would normally be carried out by a qualified social worker, who should be provided with the training, resources, time and support necessary to provide a high quality assessment. *Working Together to Safeguard Children* (HMG, 2018) outlines the qualities of a high quality assessment as shown in the box below.

. . . .

High quality assessment practice (HMG, 2018: 1:51)

High quality assessments:

- are child-centred. Where there is a conflict of interest, decisions should be made in the child's best interests: be rooted in child development: be age-appropriate; and be informed by evidence
- are focused on action and outcomes for children
- are holistic in approach, addressing the child's needs within their family and any risks the child faces from within the wider community
- ensure equality of opportunity
- involve children, ensuring that their voice is heard and provide appropriate support to enable this where the child has specific communication needs
- involve families
- identify risks to the safety and welfare of children
- build on strengths as well as identifying difficulties
- are integrated in approach
- are multi-agency and multi-disciplinary
- are a continuing process, not an event
- lead to action, including the provision of services
- review services provided on an ongoing basis.

. . . .

Assessments are complex and demanding – and will be more complex where there is more than one child in the household who requires an assessment or where the child is subject to another assessment, for example, in relation to any complex additional needs. An assessment has to take account of risk (Parton, 2010), a process which is effectively summarised in *Working Together to Safeguard Children*:

> No system can fully eliminate risk. Understanding risk involves judgment and balance. To manage risks, social workers and other practitioners should make decisions with the best interests of the child in mind, informed by the evidence available and underpinned by knowledge of child development. (HMG, 2018: 1:57)

The assessment should be based in partnership practice if at all possible; it should be evidence-based, draw on multi-agency sources and should reach informed and practical judgement of the situation. A sound assessment should be the basis of an effective plan to ensure that the best interests of the child or young person are comprehensively addressed. For social workers based in England, *Working Together to Safeguard Children* (2018) determines that within:

> one working day of a referral being received, a local authority social worker should acknowledge receipt to the referrer and make a decision about next steps and the type of response required. (HMG, 2018, 1:71)

It is further mandated that a full assessment should be undertaken within 45 days from the referral being received.

A premise of this book is that good safeguarding practice is necessarily effective multi-professional practice – at the case level and at the local leadership level. When assessments are being undertaken they can be underpinned by a number of multi-agency meetings or discussions. As outlined in *Working Together to Safeguard Children* these discussions should commence as follows:

> Strategy meetings – are intended to share information, discuss any criminal implications, whether any immediate action is required and whether a safeguarding investigation is required. The discussion – which can be face-to-face or by telephone – should include the referrer, the police, a nursery or school representative and a health professional. If the investigations warrant it then the social work manager should convene a child protection conference within 15 days of the strategy discussion. (HMG, 2018: 47)

An Initial Child Protection Conference (ICPC) is a central process in safeguarding children who are regarded having suffered or being at risk of suffering significant harm. *Working Together to Safeguard Children* (2018) describes an ICPC as follows:

Following section 47 enquiries, an initial child protection conference brings together family members (and the child where appropriate), with the supporters, advocates and practitioners most involved with the child and family, to make decisions about the child's future safety, health and development. If concerns relate to an unborn child, consideration should be given as to whether to hold a child protection conference prior to the child's birth. (HMG, 2018: 46)

The objective of the ICPC is to agree and outline a child protection plan. The aim of the plan is to ensure that the child is safe, to promote their health and development and to support the family in protecting the child.

The plan is monitored by a core group of the key practitioners working with the family. They should ensure that the plan is implemented, update the child protection plan as the situation changes, decide which professional should do what and carry out the necessary tasks. The plan should be reviewed at a Child Protection Review Conference (CPRC). This should meet within three months of the ICPC and at maximum intervals of six months thereafter. The plan can be discontinued when the child has reached 18, or dies or leaves the country, or where it is judged that the child no longer requires safeguarding.

Assessment involves a number of skills, which are outlined below:

1   Relating
2   Gathering data
3   Understanding data
4   Presenting data
5   Linking action to assessment.

Let us explore each of these skills in turn.

Relating

The assessment process should be based in the skill of relating: the ability to relate, empathise and communicate effectively. These skills can be taught and reflected upon during professional training and later in supervision. If practised to a high standard such skills will enhance the process of assessment and the quality of the assessment reports produced.

Gathering data

All professional courses will explore gathering data, perhaps through modules looking at wider research data or more focused family-based data. Data can be gathered from existing records, from work with the family and from communication with other practitioners. It is important to check all data gathered back with the family as errors in one set of professional records can often be wrongly reproduced if not double checked. This data should be situated in our wider research-based knowledge available from organisations such as *Research in Practice* or *NICE* (The National Institute for Health and Care Excellence).

Understanding data

Data in itself is not helpful unless it is interpreted and used as a guide for action: this is an important part of reflective practice and of reflection in action. The professional can ask: 'I know that x and y have happened, but what does it mean for my practice and how can this data inform my work with the family?' Again it is helpful to check against the material held by leading research organisations: for example, NICE guidance provides advice of working with parents who may have learning difficulties.

Presenting data

The presentation of data gathered during the assessment process is vital. Material should be presented in a way that is accessible to practitioners and family members alike – avoiding jargon and judgements that are not based in data.

Linking action to assessment

There are many debates about the use of such terms as 'evidence-led', 'evidence-based' and 'evidence-informed' practice. Wherever you may sit within this continuum it is important that following the assessment process your professional practice is based on sound data. The child protection plan should be based on the data gathered during the assessment process and any changes since then.

Practice point

Ask your practice educator / team manager if you can study an assessment that they regard as high quality.

Use this to learn and assist you in producing high quality assessments.

Conclusion

The aims of this chapter have been to:

- Understand the importance of family support and offering 'early help'
- Reflect on the role of assessment in safeguarding children and young people
- Consider the skills required in assessment and support practice
- Analyse the role of multi-professional working in assessment and support practice.

It has been argued in this chapter that safeguarding, except in all but the most urgent of situations, should be underpinned by family support (sometimes known as early help) in order to ensure that parents and carers are worked with in order to help them overcome any problems they may face. Where these challenges are complex, work with the family should be based on assessment: a partnership process in which practitioners should work alongside families wherever possible. Effective assessments should be embedded in multi-professional working and reflective practice.

Recommended reading

Mary Shannon, *Family Support for Social Care Practitioners* (2019)

> A well-written and wide-ranging exploration of family support aimed at social care practitioners, including an exploration of adult services. The book blends research findings, theory and practice very well.

Nick Frost and colleagues, *Family Support: Prevention, Early Intervention and Early Help* (2015)

> This book explores theory, research findings and practice in relation to family support for children, young people and their families.

John Canavan and colleagues, *Understanding Family Support: Policy, Practice and Theory* (2016)

> Written by a team that have influenced policy and practice across the Republic of Ireland and Northern Ireland this book has particular emphasis on the relation between reflective practice and family support.

6

WORKING WITH FAMILIES: CHILD ABUSE WITHIN THE FAMILY

CONTENTS

The aims of the chapter are to:

- Explore and define forms of abuse within the family
- Assess the opportunities for prevention
- Outline ways of working with families in cases of physical abuse, neglect, emotional abuse and sexual abuse within the household
- Examine multi-professional practice with households
- Explore the potential outcomes of working with families

Introduction

Most neglect, physical and emotional abuse occurs within families and households: this is the 'bread and butter' of safeguarding work and makes up the majority of social workers' and other practitioners' caseloads, although, arguably, in recent years home-based abuse has been underplayed by dramatic headlines about child sexual exploitation and other forms of contextual abuse. This chapter explores the nature of this abuse within the household and how safeguarding practitioners can work together to prevent and respond to abuse that takes place in household settings. The chapter should be read in tandem with Chapter 3 which explored underpinning theories and explanations and Chapter 9 which is focused on the skills required to work in household settings where the home visit is central.

Forms of abuse in the household

Our understanding and conceptualisation of abuse in the household has traditionally been divided into four categories:

1   Physical abuse
2   Emotional abuse
3   Neglect
4   Sexual abuse.

We will examine each of these in turn, but as we have already argued, safeguarding practice is always complex, and these four categories tend overlap and often co-exist – for example neglect, physical abuse and sexual abuse all contain elements of emotional abuse. Practitioners should always keep these interactions between different forms of abuse in mind when working in these emotionally and practically demanding situations.

Physical abuse

Incidence and prevention

Most of the high-profile Serious Case Reviews (SCRs) in England where children have died, from Maria Colwell (Field-Fisher, 1974; Jones, 2014) to Peter Connelly, have involved physical abuse and as a consequence it is an issue with a high public and political profile. It is a situation where practitioners are aware of the potentially serious consequences where things go wrong. The underlying issue that explains why this is a controversial area of practice, as we argued earlier in this book, is because it represents an interface between the State and the household, between the public arena and the privacy of the household – which is a complex space to negotiate and operate in. This area of practice is therefore very demanding of professional skills and resilience, an issue discussed more fully in Chapter 9. Physical abuse is defined in *Working Together to Safeguard Children* (HMG, 2018) as follows:

> A form of abuse which may involve hitting, shaking, throwing, poisoning, burning or scalding, drowning, suffocating or otherwise causing physical harm to a child. Physical harm may also be caused when a parent or carer fabricates the symptoms of, or deliberately induces, illness in a child. (HMG, 2018: 103)

The NSPCC found that in the UK 10.2 per cent of males and 12.9 per cent of females, aged between 18 and 24, self-reported having been severely physically abused during their childhood (NSPCC, 2018). This demonstrates the significant prevalence of this form of abuse and that practitioners are not dealing with the entire extent of abuse that takes place, given the relatively small numbers of children that become subject to child protection plans.

As with other forms of child maltreatment the physical abuse of children can and should be prevented: being engaged with prevention should always be high on professional agendas. The following points provide some guidance on prevention of physical abuse:

- Physical abuse can be prevented if we campaign, if we demonstrate awareness and intervene as appropriately and as early as possible. Methods of prevention apply to us all as practitioners and/or as parents and carers.
- Parents should seek help if they feel stressed, anxious or have violent feelings.
- Parenting skills courses can support parents in building skills and coping mechanisms.
- Children should be seen as people in their own right and not regarded as being the property of adults: phrases such as 'because I say so' should be avoided.

- Socially we should devise child-centred communities that support children and young people and support positive parenting.
- Parents with drug, alcohol or mental health problems should seek urgent and skilled help. (www.eschooltoday.com/child-abuse/physical-child-abuse/prevention-of-physical-child-abuse.html, accessed 20 April 2020).

This correctly places the physical abuse of children within the wider ecological and social context of households. Like other forms of abuse, physical abuse fundamentally reflects the abuse of power over children, it therefore relates to wider issues such as social attitudes to childhood and adult perspectives that see children as being the property of adults. This in turn links to concerns about the 'legitimated' use of the physical punishment of children and young people. There is a continuum between legitimated physical punishment and the severe physical abuse of children reported in the NSPCC survey. In 2009 the British Royal College of Paediatrics and Child Health commented on this issue as follows:

> corporal punishment of children in the home is of importance to paediatricians because of its connection with child abuse ... all paediatricians will have seen children who have been injured as a result of parental chastisement. It is not possible logically to differentiate between a smack and a physical assault since both are forms of violence. The motivation behind the smack cannot reduce the hurtful impact it has on the child. (Royal College of Paediatrics and Child Health, 2009, http://rcpch.adlibhosting.com/files/Corporal Punishment Position Statement 2009-11.pdf, accessed 21 February 2020)

The Royal College also highlighted the link with wider social factors:

> Societies which promote the needs and rights of children have a low incidence of child maltreatment, and this includes a societal rejection of physical punishment of children. (Royal College of Paediatrics and Child Health, 2009, http://rcpch.adlibhosting.com/files/Corporal%20Punishment%20Position%20Statement%202009-11.pdf, accessed 21 February 2020)

This position, taken by a highly respected professional body, makes a clear link between physical punishment within households and concerns about the physical abuse of children and young people. The organisation End Corporal Punishment (www.endcorporalpunishment.org) campaigns on this issue. They argue that:

- children and young people should be protected under the law in the same way that adults are
- the primary purpose of laws against physical punishment is educative rather than punitive

- corporal punishment is an infringement of the rights of the child under international law
- corporal punishment has a negative impact on children and young people in terms of their development
- using violence against children and young people gives the wrong message about the use of violence in general
- corporal punishment against children and young people leads to a wider use of violence in society as a whole
- the prohibition of corporal punishment raises the status of children in society and makes society a more positive and less violent environment (see https:// endcorporalpunishment.org/, accessed 6 January 2020).

We can see in the End Corporal Punishment material that there is a connection between the day-to-day violence towards children and young people and the wider concerns about the social status of childhood and youth. Where physical punishment of children in households has been banned, as in Sweden, there are indications of positive social consequences:

> There is evidence from two qualitative studies that although Swedish parents tended to be rather permissive in the early 1980s, this has changed and they now are generally quite skilled in using democratic childrearing methods. … Further, rates of child abuse appear to have declined; the number of referrals to St. Göan's Hospital in Stockholm, which receives all child maltreatment cases, had declined by 1989 to one-sixth of the 1970 rate … By the mid-1980s, Swedish rates of physical discipline and child abuse were half those found in the U.S. … and the Swedish rate of child death due to abuse was less than one-third the American rate. (Durrant, 1996: 23)

This Swedish evidence suggests that abolishing physical punishment in the home has wider positive social consequences. More recently, the Swedish lead has been followed in a variety of countries including in Scotland which passed the Children (Equal Protection from Assault) (Scotland) Act, 2019, which stated that:

> The rule of law, that the physical punishment of a child in the exercise of a parental right or a right derived from having charge or care of the child is justifiable and is therefore not an assault, ceases to have effect.

A similar position was reached in South Africa following a ruling by the Constitutional Court on 18 September 2019.

We can see therefore that our professional concerns about physical abuse in the household link with wider social and political issues.

━━━━━━━━━━━ **Reflection point** ━━━━━━━━━━━

What are your own values in relation to disciplining children you know? Which techniques would you prefer in relation to discipline?

Are there disciplinary methods you object to?

How do these personal values and attitudes relate to your professional practice?

Safeguarding children from physical abuse

We now move on more specifically to safeguarding children from physical abuse within the household and the role of safeguarding practitioners in doing this. We can locate the start of modern understandings in the work of Henry Kempe, and his promotion of the concept of 'battered baby syndrome', after which physical abuse became a key focus of professional practice and later of public concern (see Kempe et al., 2013). Kempe himself reflects as follows:

> I coined the term 'The Battered Child Syndrome', in 1962, despite its provocative and anger-producing nature. I had for the preceding ten years talked about child abuse, non-accidental, or inflicted injury, but few paid attention. At a gathering very much like this in 1962, describing in some detail the physical findings, both subtle and severe, of the battered child and at the same time beginning to point out some of the dynamics involved in child abuse, there did result a degree of public attention. (Kempe, 1971: 28)

We can note here the wider context that those who have attempted to raise the profile of child abuse – including Sigmund Freud, Henry Kempe and in Cleveland (England) in 1988, Marietta Higgs – all faced public criticism when they disclosed the nature and extent of different forms of child abuse.

Physical abuse has featured strongly in many high-profile child deaths reports including those relating to Maria Colwell, Tyra Henry, Kimberley Carlile, Jasmine Beckford, Victoria Climbié and Peter Connelly (Jones, 2014). This profile has declined as, since the turn of the twenty-first century, there has been more focus on child sexual abuse and exploitation. It is possible that the profile of physical abuse will again increase if another tragic child death features in the media. Referrals about physical abuse are always prominent within child protection systems.

Practitioners, particularly those within schools and day care settings, need to be aware of the signs of potential abuse. It is not their role to provide a 'diagnosis' – this will be carried out by paediatricians, who have expertise in assessing the causes of bruises and other injuries. All safeguarding practitioners have to be aware of is when physical abuse may be occurring. For example, bruised knees are usually part of the day-to-day rough and tumble of childhood: bruises on the arm which resemble adult finger prints clearly are not. It is important to listen to children's accounts of what has happened – whilst remembering that they may be scared or reluctant to tell the truth. Some injuries may be life threatening and this is when urgent action to remove the child may be required – an Emergency Protection Order or Police Protection Order under the Children Act 1989, for example. Other injuries may be less serious, and the professional actions will often depend on the parental responses: a regretful and cooperative parent can be worked with; a parent in denial or aggression from parents will make it harder for practitioners to devise an effective family support or safeguarding plan. Carrying out a comprehensive multi-professional assessment will allow practitioners to form an evidence-informed judgement in relation to a specific incident.

Practice point

When working with cases of suspected or actual physical harm you should consider:

Is a full assessment required?

What are the strengths in the household you could work with?

What is the attitude of the parent/carer? Are they cooperative and responding to the issues you raise? Beware of 'disguised compliance' (as in the Baby Peter case where the mother seemed to be cooperative but in actual fact was not).

Has the child said anything that causes you concern?

Is there a medical assessment of the injuries? What can you learn from this?

Have you considered creative forms of direct work with the child – using visual techniques for example?

Emotional abuse of children and young people

Incidence and prevention

Whereas physical abuse will usually result in visible signs, even if these are sometimes hard to interpret, the occurrence of emotional abuse is more difficult to perceive. Emotional abuse will usually occur in the privacy of the household and the impact will be difficult to assess. The emotional abuse of children is defined in *Working Together to Safeguard Children* (HMG, 2018) as follows:

> The persistent emotional maltreatment of a child such as to cause severe and persistent adverse effects on the child's emotional development. It may involve conveying to a child that they are worthless or unloved, inadequate, or valued

only insofar as they meet the needs of another person. It may include not giving the child opportunities to express their views, deliberately silencing them or 'making fun' of what they say or how they communicate. It may feature age or developmentally inappropriate expectations being imposed on children. These may include interactions that are beyond a child's developmental capability, as well as overprotection and limitation of exploration and learning, or preventing the child participating in normal social interaction. It may involve seeing or hearing the ill-treatment of another. It may involve serious bullying (including cyber bullying), causing children frequently to feel frightened or in danger, or the exploitation or corruption of children. Some level of emotional abuse is involved in all types of maltreatment of a child, though it may occur alone. (HMG, 2018: 104)

We should also mention that emotional abuse is linked to a child or young person witnessing domestic abuse. Emotional abuse is both complex and difficult to assess. Whilst most emotional abuse will occur 'behind closed doors' we will all recall hearing a child being told to 'shut up' or being told to do something because 'I say so' in a supermarket or on public transport. These are examples of emotional abuse and therefore of children and young people being regarded as the property of adults and of being under-valued as both individuals and as a social group. The box below outlines some of the features that make up emotional abuse.

· ·

Emotional abuse includes

- humiliating or constantly criticising a child
- threatening, shouting at a child or calling them names
- making the child the subject of jokes, or using sarcasm to hurt a child
- blaming and scapegoating
- making a child perform degrading acts
- not recognising a child's own individuality or trying to control their lives
- pushing a child too hard or not recognising their limitations
- exposing a child to upsetting events or situations, like domestic abuse or drug taking
- failing to promote a child's social development
- not allowing them to have friends
- persistently ignoring them
- being absent
- manipulating a child
- never saying anything kind, expressing positive feelings or congratulating a child on successes
- never showing any emotions in interactions with a child, also known as emotional neglect.

(Reproduced with the kind permission of the NSPCC. www.nspcc.org.UK/what-is-child-abuse/types-of-abuse/emotional-abuse/#types,accessed 6 February 2020)

· ·

Emotional abuse is both widespread and diverse in the forms it takes. All the factors identified above demonstrate a lack of empathy for the child: a failure to see the world from the perspective of the child or young person. Just as we stated in relation to physical abuse earlier in this chapter, the emotional abuse of children and young people is part of a mind-set that sees children as the property of parents and not as full human beings in their own right. Some prominent commentators, such as Anthony Giddens and Harry Ferguson, have argued for more democratic family forms in order that children are treated more equally within households.

Children who are victims of emotional abuse do not experience any form of 'crazy love', the term used by Bronfenbrenner earlier in this book, or the dedicated care that will help them grow into strong and confident adults. It is surprising that most modern Western States are still a long way from having universal parenting preparation programmes which would enable parents to be aware of powerful and important messages, such as that provided by Bronfenbrenner (Frost et al., 2015).

Reflection point

How could children that you know, professionally or personally, be treated with more respect and involved more in decision-making in the home?

Think of a time you have witnessed a child being shouted at or verbally abused in a public setting such as in a supermarket. Did you intervene? When would a situation be so serious that you would intervene? What would you say to a parent/carer who has been emotionally abusive to a child? What are the barriers to intervening?

Working with emotional abuse

As with our discussion of physical abuse, emotional abuse has a wider social significance and is connected with specific factors that practitioners will have to deal with on a day-to-day basis, which includes a clear link with domestic abuse. The box below outlines some of the factors that the professional may come across and which may raise concerns about the existence of emotional abuse.

Signs of emotional abuse

There might not be any obvious physical signs of emotional abuse or neglect. And a child might not tell anyone what's happening until they reach a 'crisis point'. That's why it's important to look out for signs in how a child is acting.

As children grow up, their emotions change. This means it can be difficult to tell if they're being emotionally abused. But children who are being emotionally abused might:

(Continued)

- seem unconfident or lack self-assurance
- struggle to control their emotions
- have difficulty making or maintaining relationships
- act in a way that's inappropriate for their age.

If a child reveals abuse

A child who is being emotionally abused might not realise what's happening is wrong. And they might even blame themselves. If a child talks to you about emotional abuse it's important to:

- listen carefully to what they're saying
- let them know they've done the right thing by telling you
- tell them it's not their fault
- say you'll take them seriously
- don't confront the alleged abuser
- explain what you'll do next
- report what the child has told you as soon as possible.

(Reproduced with the kind permission of the NSPCC. www.nspcc.org.UK/what-is-child-abuse/types-of-abuse/emotional-abuse/#signs, accessed 7 January 2020)

The child who experiences emotional abuse may well grow up to be an adult who feels unloved, self-blaming and lacking in self-confidence. It is important therefore that practitioners take action to support such children. Any action should be based in:

- Careful direct work and observation of the child
- Talking to the parent about parenting and helping a child to feel valued and loved
- Well-planned multi-disciplinary assessment, with a nominated lead professional in place
- Detailed consideration of what is in the best interests of the child.

With well-timed and appropriate professional support, or at the extreme in an alternative care placement, the child should be supported to build their self-confidence and self-esteem. Drawing on Bronfenbrenner's argument (1991), discussed earlier in this book, they may well display the resilience to overcome adverse childhood experiences: particularly when they have a significant figure in their lives who provides consistent warmth and care.

Practice point

Many children experience emotional abuse: how would you define 'significant harm' in relation to emotional abuse?

You may wish to consider the following points:

- persistent and regular emotional abuse by parents or carers
- a child who is demonstrating low self-esteem
- a child who has issues in relating to others
- a child who is self-harming.

Sexual abuse in the household

Incidence and prevention

Sexual abuse is perhaps the most profound social challenge of all the forms of abuse explored here. The sexual abuse of both adults and children has led to social protest movements across the world, such as the #MeToo movement which began in Hollywood and mass protests against rape in India (Raj and McDougal, 2014). As with other forms of abuse, sexual abuse raises wider social issues about power, gender and exploitation which are explored in more depth in Chapters 4 and 7 of this book.

The sexual abuse of children is defined in *Working Together to Safeguard Children* (HMG, 2018) as involving:

> forcing or enticing a child or young person to take part in sexual activities, not necessarily involving a high level of violence, whether or not the child is aware of what is happening. The activities may involve physical contact, including assault by penetration (for example, rape or oral sex) or non-penetrative acts such as masturbation, kissing, rubbing and touching outside of clothing. They may also include non-contact activities, such as involving children in looking at, or in the production of, sexual images, watching sexual activities, encouraging children to behave in sexually inappropriate ways, or grooming a child in preparation for abuse. Sexual abuse can take place online, and technology can be used to facilitate offline abuse. Sexual abuse is not solely perpetrated by adult males. Women can also commit acts of sexual abuse, as can other children. (HMG, 2018: 104)

In 2017 the NSPCC reported that 5.1 per cent of males and 17.8 per cent of females aged 18–24 reported sexual abuse involving some form of contact during their childhood (NSPCC, 2017). Kelly and Karsna (2017) point out that this suggests that safeguarding agencies are responding to only a small proportion of this incidence. They demonstrate that whilst the number of children subject to a child protection plan for sexual abuse in England and Wales has stayed relatively stable at around 3,000 at any given time, the police recorded over 53,000 sexual offences against children in just one year. There is clearly a significant gap between the actual incidence of child sexual abuse and safeguarding practitioners' responses to it. Safeguarding practitioners should hold this in mind in their practice: we are, collectively, not responding adequately to the full extent of child sexual abuse: the Savile case study in Chapter 4 provides an example of this and what the explanations may be.

One reason for the low rate of response to child sexual abuse may be that sexual abuse in the family is one of those unthinkable events that calls for skilled and insightful professional work and which also highlights why 'common sense' approaches do not apply in safeguarding practice. There has long been a taboo against sexual abuse in the family – often labelled with the term 'incest'. Most societies have had an incest taboo – often overseen and policed by religious organisations. It is surprising that incest did not become illegal in the United Kingdom until the passage of the Punishment of Incest Act, in 1908 (Bell, 2002). There are profound social and psychological reasons why collectively we have been in denial about the extent of child sexual abuse.

Whilst the *Working Together to Safeguard Children* definition, quoted earlier, is strictly accurate, the final two sentences are in danger of giving a false impression as the vast majority of sexual abuse is perpetrated by males, and any given professional is very unlikely to come across a female perpetrator. As we can see from the NSPCC statistics, quoted earlier, females are most likely to be victims and perpetrators are more likely to be male. Sexual abuse is profoundly a gendered phenomenon.

Feminists have campaigned for many decades against the sexual abuse of women and girls – this emerged as campaigns against rape and sexual abuse following the feminist movements of the 1960s, and in recent decades has become more high profile following the #MeToo movement, campaigning initially against abuse by Hollywood film producers. Sexual abuse is a dominant force in society which helps to shape day-to-day interactions between all men and women: it has an impact, for example, on the freedom of women to move around towns and cities. Prevention of sexual abuse therefore raises fundamental challenges for society: the existence of sexual assault by males leads to issues about how we raise boys and how we perceive masculinity (see: www.theguardian.com/world/2018/mar/12/masculinity-gender-men-sexual-assault-rape, accessed 16 February 2020).

More specifically in relation to childhood and sexual abuse the NSPCC have organised an effective prevention campaign – known as PANTS (www.nspcc.org.UK/keeping-children-safe/support-for-parents/underwear-rule/).

The focus of the campaign is on the prevention of child sexual abuse, using the principles outlined below.

Principles of the **NSPCC PANTS** campaign

Privates are private

Always remember your body belongs to you

No means no

Talk about secrets that upset you

Speak up, someone can help

(Reproduced with the kind permission of the NSPCC. www.nspcc.org.uk/keeping-children-safe/support-for-parents/underwear-rule/, accessed 20 April 2020)

The campaign provides learning materials for a variety of audiences. The box below provides the learning objectives for teachers who are able to utilise the materials.

Learning objectives of the **NSPCC PANTS** campaign

Children will be able to:

- understand and learn the PANTS rules
- name body parts and know which parts should be private
- know the difference between appropriate and inappropriate touch
- understand that they have the right to say 'no' to unwanted touch
- start thinking about who they trust and who they can ask for help.

(Reproduced with the kind permission of the NSPCC.)

Further guidance on the prevention of child sexual abuse, using a wider lens, is provided below.

There are many other elements to preventing sexual abuse which can sit alongside initiatives such as the PANTS campaign. The official US Child Welfare site highlights the following:

- The responsibility sits with adults, but it is also important to give all the protective tools they require
- Adults should be involved in children's lives and know who their children are mixing with – including on the internet
- Be aware of grooming techniques from adults the child knows: such as trying to be alone with the child, or giving inappropriate gifts
- Making sure that organisations and groups that your child is involved with follow safe care practices – including staff and volunteer recruitment

- Make it possible for your children or children you know to talk to you about difficult subjects, including the difference between good secrets and bad secrets
- In keeping with the PANTS campaign ensure children know about okay touch and inappropriate touch
- Make sure children are empowered to make their own decisions about their own bodies
- Pursue any issues that make you feel uncomfortable – for example about the behaviour of other adults
- If your child or a child you know discloses to you – respond calmly and supportively.

(www.childwelfare.gov/pubPDFs/prevent_sa_ts.pdf, accessed 7 January 2020)

Related to these campaigns to prevent child sexual abuse there have been movements for improving therapy and support for victims and survivors: at the time of writing this book this is probably the most significant shortfall in terms of service provision for victims and survivors of sexual abuse. In an interview-based study by the current author it is argued that in relation to child sexual exploitation:

It also emerges from the interviews that whereas the practitioners feel able to offer support and effective multi-disciplinary interventions, there are still many challenges and barriers in offering effective longer-term, mental health interventions. There is, the respondents suggest, a serious challenge for public mental health resulting from the shortfall in service provision for young people's mental health. (Frost, 2019: 43)

The Courage to Heal written by Ellen Bass and Laura Davis (1988) was a landmark therapeutic text whose main message was that the victim/survivor was clearly not to blame when sexual abuse had taken place. Individual or group therapy can play a key role in turning a 'victim' into a 'survivor', the latter being the preferred term for people who have experienced abuse and managed to move on and who do not want to be defined by their abusive experiences.

Reflection point

To what extent is the sexual abuse of children rooted in everyday attitudes to gender and gender difference?

How can your profession contribute to the prevention of sexual abuse and sexual assault in society?

Safeguarding children from child sexual abuse in the household

Sexual abuse is a serious and damaging occurrence which can leave victims and survivors deeply psychologically scarred, particularly if adequate support is not provided. When sexual abuse occurs within the family or household there is an additional dynamic which is complex and has a profound impact on victims. For example, if the perpetrator is the father, the child may feel dependent on the father and have the usual feelings of love and affection. The father may have exploited these feelings as part of a grooming process. The dynamic is therefore complicated: the child may feel guilt and a sense of self-blame. In addition, the mother often feels a sense of letting the child down. When a number of footballers in England spoke about being sexually abused by their coaches they linked the difficulty of disclosing to parents to the ambitions of parents in relation to football and that this made disclosure about so-called 'role models' more difficult (Taylor, 2017). This is illustrative of the complex dynamics unleashed by the sexual abuse of children, both within and outside of the household setting.

The practitioner needs to be aware of these dynamics when they intervene. For example, if the child is removed from the household to protect them then this may well give a message that the child is to blame and that removal can be seen as a form of punishment.

As with other forms of abuse we need to be wary of checklists, but there are signs of sexual abuse which all practitioners should be aware of. These include, for example:

- Unexplained injuries, pain or soreness in the genital or anal area
- Sudden onset of worries, depression, nightmares or bedwetting
- Withdrawn or anti-social behaviour
- Loss of appetite or unusual eating patterns
- Unexplained avoidance of certain places, people or events
- Surprising or inappropriate sexualised behaviour or knowledge.

(See www.childwelfare.gov/pubPDFs/prevent_sa_ts.pdf, accessed 7 January 2020)

Working with child sexual abuse within the household will require all the skills discussed in Chapter 9 – practitioners will always find this work demanding both personally and professionally. The US organisation RAINN (Rape, Abuse and Incest National Network) makes the following useful suggestions for talking to a child that may have been sexually abused.

Talking to a child about sexual abuse

- **Pick your time and place carefully**. Choose a space where the child is comfortable or ask them where they'd like to talk. Avoid talking in front of someone who may be causing the harm.
- **Be aware of your tone**. If you start the conversation in a serious tone, you may scare the child, and they may be more likely to give you the answers they think you want to hear – rather than the truth. Try to make the conversation more casual. A non-threatening tone will help put the child at ease and ultimately provide you with more accurate information.
- **Talk to the child directly**. Ask questions that use the child's own vocabulary, but that are a little vague. For example, "Has someone been touching you?" In this context "touching" can mean different things, but it is likely a word the child is familiar with. The child can respond with questions or comments to help you better gauge the situation like, "No one touches me except my mom at bath time," or "You mean like the way my cousin touches me sometimes?" Understand that sexual abuse can feel good to the child, so asking if someone is "hurting" them may not bring out the information that you are looking for.
- **Listen and follow up.** Allow the child to talk freely. Wait for them to pause, and then follow up on points that made you feel concerned.
- **Avoid judgment and blame**. Avoid placing blame by using "I" questions and statements. Rather than beginning your conversation by saying, "You said something that made me worry…" consider starting your conversation with the word "I." For example: "I am concerned because I heard you say that you are not allowed to sleep in your bed by yourself."
- **Reassure the child**. Make sure that the child knows that they are not in trouble. Let them know you are simply asking questions because you are concerned about them.
- **Be patient**. Remember that this conversation may be very frightening for the child. Many perpetrators make threats about what will happen if someone finds out about the abuse. They may tell a child that they will be put into foster care or threaten them or their loved ones with physical violence.

(Reproduced with the kind permission of RAINN. https://www.rainn.org/articles/if-you-suspect-child-being-harmed)

Whilst these tips are written for a parent, or other concerned adult, they also work well for practitioners.

If, following the initial interview process, practitioners are still concerned, they should follow their agency procedure and ensure at the more formal stages that they follow the excellent guidance provided by the British Ministry of Justice in their publication *Achieving Best Evidence in Criminal Proceedings* (Ministry of Justice, 2011). It is not possible to give an adequate account of this 250 page document in this context, but for example, it provides the following guidance in relation to asking open questions:

An open-ended question is the best kind of question from the point of view of information gathering (i.e. gaining good quality information). Therefore, this type of question should be used predominantly during the interview. Open-ended questions are framed in such a way that the witness is able to give an unrestricted answer, which in turn enables the witness to control the flow of information in the interview. This questioning style also minimises the risk that the interviewer will impose their view of what happened on the witness. Questions beginning with the phrase 'Tell me' or the word 'Describe' are useful examples of this type of question, e.g. 'You said you were in the shopping centre this morning when something happened, tell me everything that you can remember.' (Ministry of Justice, 2011: para. 3.45–6)

The practitioner should follow their own organisation's code of conduct, and allow free narrative without interruption, not asking direct questions, remain neutral, not show any emotion or encouragement other than to say 'I'm listening' and at the end to say 'Thank you'.

This guidance, whilst aimed at those conducting specialist evidential interviewing, is useful in professional practice with children more generally.

Practice point

If you know or suspect a child is experiencing sexual abuse in the family, you need to reflect carefully before talking to the child. Make sure you carefully consider the points outlined in the previous box.

Your professional role in relation to child sexual abuse is vital – you may well play a crucial role in helping improve the lives of children facing extremely distressing life situations. You will need support from the full range of practitioners to form a 'team around the child' – including social workers, health practitioners, teachers, police and therapists.

Child neglect in the household

Incidence and prevention

The neglect of children is a widespread social problem which has ramifications more widely than the day-to-day concerns of practitioners. Neglect is closely related to social issues such as poverty and inequality: in unequal societies children are foremost amongst the victims of the consequences of inequality (Wilkinson and Pickett, 2009). This section on neglect draws extensively on the work of Jan Horwath, who has been influential in developing our understanding of the issue.

Neglect is defined in *Working Together to Safeguard Children* (HMG, 2018) as follows:

> The persistent failure to meet a child's basic physical and/or psychological needs, likely to result in the serious impairment of the child's health or development. Neglect may occur during pregnancy as a result of maternal substance abuse. Once a child is born, neglect may involve a parent or carer failing to:
>
> a   provide adequate food, clothing and shelter (including exclusion from home or abandonment)
>
> b   protect a child from physical and emotional harm or danger
>
> c   ensure adequate supervision (including the use of inadequate caregivers)
>
> d   ensure access to appropriate medical care or treatment.
>
> It may also include neglect of, or unresponsiveness to, a child's basic emotional needs. (HMG, 2018: 104)

The NSPCC reported that 7 per cent of males and 11 per cent of females, aged 18–24, self-reported that they had been neglected during their childhood (NSPCC, 2017).

Neglect is perhaps the most difficult of the forms of abuse for practitioners to identify and react to. Teachers and health visitors, amongst others, often complain that the children's social care threshold is too high in relation to neglect and that social workers do not respond in the way that other practitioners may wish. Neglect is difficult to identify in terms of levels of severity and the length of time it has continued for. In low income communities, where most safeguarding work is located (Bywaters et al., 2016b), practitioners will become familiar with the impact of poverty: poor standards of nutrition, clothing and accommodation. As Brandon et al. comment in relation to Serious Case Reviews:

> This was the first of our six consecutive national analyses where poverty featured prominently in SCRs, particularly in the neglect cases. There are ongoing debates about the links between poverty and maltreatment but most studies find a correlation rather than a clear causal relationship between poverty, neglect and abuse. (2020: 273)

As a result of the impact of poverty it may then become difficult to identify the actual impact of neglect. Complex cultural judgements may also be involved where practitioners are working in multi-cultural communities (Bernard, 2019b). As we have stated before in this book, there is no easy solution to these challenges – aside from making well-informed professional judgements based in relationship-based work with the family and fundamentally embedded in effective multi-professional work.

To what degree do you regard child neglect as a social structural issue?

Is it ethical to judge parents living in poverty for the impact of poverty on their children?

How can we distinguish between the impact of poverty and neglect?

Safeguarding children from neglect

A practitioner may come across neglect in a variety of forms which can be classified as follows: emotional, disorganised, depressed or passive, and severe deprivation (Horwath and Platt, 2019).

Emotional neglect can involve actions by parents or inactions, such as ignoring the needs of the child. Parents may scapegoat the child for family problems and seek help for a 'troublesome' child. Parents may be reluctant to accept practitioner involvement and can be resistant and difficult to engage.

Disorganised neglect may occur in families that are labelled as 'problem families' and be well known to agencies. Household conditions may be chaotic and even unhygienic. Workers may find it easier to work on presenting material issues, such as shortage of clothing, but need to be aware of underlying issues as well.

Depressed or passive neglect is characterised by low energy passivity and often results in children being dirty and smelly, an issue often picked up by early years or school staff. Such families require motivation and support to overcome the very serious challenges they face.

The severe deprivation type of neglect is probably rarer and has the most profound impact on the children: their physical and emotional development may be profoundly harmed. The practitioner would notice poor social presentation, dirty home conditions and related smells. It will be hard to engage with some parents and will involve sustained and skilful practice (see www.safeguardingsheffieldchildren.org/assets/1/a_day_in_the_life_guidance.pdf, accessed 7 January 2020).

The practitioner can use a range of tools to support their practice and assess which, if any, of these categories a neglect situation may fall into. Practical tools are particularly helpful in the field of neglect which is difficult to assess and respond appropriately to. Calderdale Safeguarding Children Partnership (CSCP), for example, have drawn on the work of Horwath who produced a tool kit to assist practitioners in cases of known or suspected neglect. The Assessment of Neglect Tool incorporates *The Graded Care Profile* (Horwath and Platt, 2019) and *Home Conditions* tool and 'can be used by a wide range of practitioners, in different settings for the identification and assessment of neglect and to support a consistent, effective and integrated early response to neglected children and young people'. The tools have been developed to identify strengths as well as difficulties:

> Focussing on strengths assists the assessor to realistically assess the potential for sustained change and improvement within the family. Organising examples of evidence and analysing the impact on the child will help to clarify thresholds and identify specific approaches to work with different types of neglect. (Calderdale Safeguarding Children Partnership)

Neglect by parents may be rooted in social structural factors – such as poverty and social exclusion. It may also be related to what seem more individual and particular factors such as poor parenting skills, mental health or substance abuse challenges. These situations are complex for practitioners to change or challenge – particularly if there are combinations of, say, domestic violence, mental ill-health and substance abuse: colloquially known as the 'toxic trio' (Broadley, 2019).

Child neglect has a negative impact on children and can lead to both physical and psychological disadvantage. It can also be a long-term challenge for children and may go on for years without professional intervention. By using the *Assessment of Neglect* tool the professional can reflect upon the type of neglect the child is experiencing. Of course, as with the other forms of abuse we have discussed, it is improbable that any neglect will fall into any single category. Indeed neglect may well overlap with physical abuse, sexual abuse or emotional abuse. What is important is that an assessment of neglect leads to specific, tailored responses from the practitioners working together in the best interest of the child: again the assessment triangle works well in conceptualising and undertaking a full assessment (Horwath, 2007).

The professional needs to explore recurring issues in the child's lived experience, and work out whether the parents have the willingness and ability to change. Professional judgement should be based on the specific assessment, research and relevant theoretical perspectives (Horwath and Platt, 2019). The CSCP describe the purpose of their tool kit as follows:

> In order to fully understand how various aspects of neglect are impacting on the child, the associated risks, their unmet needs and areas of resilience, it is important to understand what life is like for them on a daily basis, at weekends, holidays and when different people care for them. In order to understand how the behaviours, attitude and parenting style of the adult contribute to the risks or unmet needs, it is also necessary to understand a day in the life of the parent/s. One way of doing this is to work with the child and the parent (separately and together) using clocks to describe what is happening for them at

different times of the day and night. The experience of a pre-verbal child or child with limited language skills or levels of understanding may need to be explored in different ways, for example, via, a pictorial timetable of their day (PECS – Pictorial Exchange Communication System), observations, specific questions with the carer about routine, mealtimes, bedtimes, etc. (Calderdale Safeguarding Children Partnership)

The purpose of 'A Day in the Life' of the child is to establish an understanding of the child's day as outlined in Table 6.1.

Table 6.1 A day in the life of the child

Morning routines and parental involvement	Child or other's responsibility for tasks, personal hygiene, dressing and availability of relevant equipment, clothes, availability of breakfast, preparation for nursery/school, appropriate parental supervision, mode of transport to nursery/school, etc.
Out of the house	Journey to and from nursery/school; relationships with others; child's presentation, e.g. tired, hungry; activities during the day; feelings associated with different people, places, activities; others' expectations, etc.
Evening routines and parental involvement	Availability of parent; availability of meals; child's responsibility for tasks, self-care, personal hygiene and availability of relevant equipment; appropriate parental supervision; access to leisure activities, friends and resources; favourite pastimes, what happens? Who is in the house? Arrangements for going to bed, etc.
Night time	Where the child sleeps; sleep patterns, disruptions; facilities etc. Who else is in the house?
Weekends and holidays	What happens? Who is involved, meals, routines and explored as above.

As we discussed, when reflecting on child sexual abuse, open questions are usually the most appropriate to explore the child's day. Suitable questions may include:

'What happens when you get home from school?'

'What is your favourite part of the day?'

'What happens at bedtime?'

'What would you like to change about your usual day?'

A similar exercise can be undertaken with parents – so that the different narratives can be compared and contrasted. The exercise allows the professional to talk to all parties about their experience and what can change.

The CSCP, drawing on the work of Horwath, suggest that final steps are to:

- look for patterns within the child and family's life;
- assess the extent to which the parents' ability/capacity to change is linked with the child's developmental needs and pace of development;
- explore alternative explanations for what is happening;
- consider what would a day in the life of this child look like if their needs were being met and risks removed;
- and finally, make professional judgements based on research, specialist knowledge and theory in order to arrive at a conclusion. (Calderdale Safeguarding Children Partnership)

A family support-based approach may well work to address neglect, but in extreme cases care proceedings may be required.

Practice point

Consider the tool kit provided by Calderdale Safeguarding Children Partnership, based on the work of Horwath, in the last part of this chapter. Explore the website of your own locality partnership to see if there are any tools that you may find useful.

Working with domestic abuse

When children and young people witness domestic violence this is child abuse: this was recognised legally in 2002 in the Adoption and Children Act, which clarifies the definition of harm contained in the Children Act 1989 in order to make it clear that the harm to a child includes the impairment of the child's health or development as a result of witnessing the ill-treatment of another person. The NSPCC outlines the psychological impact of this form of abuse as follows:

- aggression and challenging behaviour
- depression
- anxiety – including worrying about a parent's safety
- changes in mood
- difficulty interacting with others
- withdrawal
- fearfulness, including fear of conflict
- suicidal thoughts or feelings.

(Reproduced with the kind permission of the NSPCC. https://learning.nspcc.org.UK/ child-abuse-and-neglect/domestic-abuse/#heading-top, accessed 20 February 2020)

Learning from SCRs suggests that domestic abuse that later leads to child deaths is linked to the following:

- Parental mental health problems
- Substance abuse
- A history of male violence
- Young mothers may be particularly vulnerable
- Lack of take up of services
- Differing cultural norms
- Trigger events that lead to violence. (NSPCC, 2013)

A particularly disturbing analysis was carried out by Hilary Saunders, on behalf of Women's Aid Federation of England, and is graphically entitled *Twenty-Nine Child Homicides* (2004). This important report concludes that:

- In three cases it is clear that not only did the court grant orders for unsupervised contact or residence to very violent fathers but that these decisions were made against professional advice, without waiting for professional advice or without requesting professional advice. There was nothing to indicate that any court practitioners have been held accountable.
- It is clear that domestic violence was involved in 11 out of the 13 families. In one of the two remaining cases the mother has spoken of her ex-partner's obsessively controlling behaviour (a characteristic feature of domestic violence) and in the other case there were concerns about the child's safety.
- Several of the homicides occurred during overnight stays.
- Mental health issues (including depression and suicide threats or attempts) are mentioned with regard to 9 of the 13 fathers who killed their children.
- In several cases where statutory agencies knew that the mother was experiencing domestic violence, the children were not viewed as being at risk of 'significant harm', even when she was facing potentially lethal violence.
- In five cases it is clear that the father killed the children in order to take revenge on his ex-partner for leaving him.
- Some practitioners clearly did not have any understanding of the power and control dynamics of domestic violence, and did not recognise the increased risks following separation or the mother's starting a new relationship.
- In several cases practitioners did not talk to the children and this meant that, in effect, there was no assessment of their needs. Sometimes this was because the perpetrator prevented any meaningful contact with the child. (Saunders, 2004: 4–5)

Domestic violence is a frequent occurrence and in the extreme can end in child homicide. In order to address some of these serious shortcomings in service provision the NSPCC suggests that practitioners should:

Have a clear understanding of the role of men

See the mother alone

Avoid over reliance on the mother's ability to protect children

See the bigger picture

Maintain a healthy amount of scepticism

Communicate across agencies

Understand the complex nature of relationships in domestic abuse situations

Understand the impact on children and young people

Help mothers to understand the impact of domestic abuse. (NSPCC, 2018)

It should be remembered that domestic abuse can also occur between young people. For example, it has been estimated that one in four teenage girls had been hit by a boyfriend and over 30 per cent of young women have experienced sexual assault by a boyfriend (North Yorkshire County Council, 2014: 11). The North Yorkshire document suggests ways of promoting healthy relationships as outlined in the box below.

....

Promoting healthy relationships

All practitioners when working with young people have a responsibility to discuss and challenge views on:

- Assumptions, beliefs and attitudes about gender and power
- Beliefs and attitudes about men and women
- Stereotypical portrayals of gender in the media (particularly with the 'hyper-sexualisation' of the media)
- Stereotypes around domestic abuse such as the belief that the victim is 'asking for it'
- How to manage feelings and accept responsibility for one's own feelings and behaviour
- How to resolve conflict effectively
- Knowing the difference between abusive and non-abusive relationships
- Recognising that abuse is never acceptable and is a crime. (NYCC, 2014: 11. Reproduced with the kind permission of the North Yorkshire Safeguarding Children Partnership)

....

Conclusion

The aims of the chapter have been to:

- Explore and define forms of abuse within the family
- Assess the opportunities for prevention

- Outline ways of working with families in cases of physical abuse, neglect, emotional abuse and sexual abuse within the household
- Examine multi-professional practice with households
- Explore the potential outcomes of working with families.

Throughout this book we have written about effective safeguarding work being relationship-based, building on well-informed assessments and working together with other practitioners. Theoretically, working with families is complex as it represents the interface between the State (in the form of local practitioners and court systems) and the private realm of the household. Negotiating this boundary through professional practices such as the home visit and the child protection conference is demanding and difficult work. This chapter has attempted to provide practical insights for the practitioners confronted with child abuse in their everyday practice.

Recommended reading

Ray Jones, *The Story of Baby P* (2014)

Jones provides an excellent account of this high-profile English child death – addressing both practice issues and the wider social context, including the reasons for the case becoming politically high-profile.

Sarah Nelson, *Tackling Child Sexual Abuse* (2016)

An excellent, comprehensive account of understanding and opposing child sexual abuse. Nelson explores both the social context and the impact of abuse on individuals as both children and adults.

Jadwiga Leigh and Jane Laing, *Thinking about Child Protection Practice* (2018)

This book is fully embedded in practice – using case studies from the experience of the authors and sharing their reflections on practice.

7

UNDERSTANDING CHILD SEXUAL EXPLOITATION

CONTENTS

The aims of this chapter are to:

- Explain and analyse the impact of child sexual exploitation
- Understand the role of the professional in relation to 'contextual safeguarding'
- Reflect on the changing nature of safeguarding policy and practice

Introduction

The next two chapters aim to explore child abuse that takes place within and across localities – rather than that which largely takes place within the household. The focus in this chapter is on child sexual exploitation (CSE) which has been the highest profile safeguarding issue in the UK thus far during the twenty-first century. Having explored CSE specifically, the following chapter moves on to examine the more recent shift towards 'contextual safeguarding' which provides a wider understanding of how this issue relates to other forms of exploitation, including modern slavery, gangs and 'county lines'.

Understanding child sexual exploitation

Throughout this book we have reflected on how the safeguarding process is socially constructed and how, as a result, new forms of understanding have emerged and consequently professional approaches have changed. There is no clearer example of this process than the phenomenon known as child sexual exploitation. Since around the year 2000 in the UK we have moved from having very little grasp or understanding of CSE (approximately 2000 until 2010), to a crisis period where CSE emerged to become a high-profile public issue and was named as a 'national emergency' (2010 until 2015), with the almost inevitable criticism of practitioners, and then forward to the contemporary more pro-active, comprehensive and strategic approach. After about 2015 CSE came to be seen in a wider context and understanding has developed around the concept of 'contextual safeguarding', a shift which is explored in Chapter 8. In this chapter we begin with an exploration of CSE and then go on to analyse how the move to contextual safeguarding emerged: we also explore the skills and approaches required by practitioners in relation to this. The current state of policy and practice will be outlined and analysed.

Child sexual exploitation: A lack of understanding and subsequent poor policy responses

As discussed earlier in this book (see Chapter 1) the sexual exploitation of children has probably existed for as long as human history. For long periods of history the sexual abuse of children was not seen as a crime and was not seen as in any way exploitative. There is no doubt that CSE has existed throughout the centuries, but we did not have the language, values or concepts formed to fully understand it. It is significant that Rachel Feinstein calls her book about sexual assault and slavery, *When Rape was Legal: The Untold History of Sexual Violence During Slavery* (2018). A further example comes from the journalist W.T. Stead (1885) who wrote a notorious article entitled 'The Maiden Tribute of Modern Babylon' in a popular magazine, the *Pall Mall Gazette*. Stead described how a 'maiden' could be purchased for £5 in a way which we would now name and understand as CSE (Robinson, 2012).

In preparing this text the author has attempted to research the origins of the key terms. It seems that the book written by Judith Ennew, *The Sexual Exploitation of Children* (1986), was the first to use the term 'sexual exploitation'. She utilises the idea of 'exploitation' to explore the global sexual abuse of children, with a particular focus on 'sex tourism'. Ennew theorises her approach by exploring the abuse of power and she researches the factors that generate inequality of power – gender, social class, ethnicity and geography (to this we should add disability; Miller and Brown, 2014). Ennew argues that major power differentials exist between wealthy, white, Western men in contrast to poor black or Asian girls in, for example, the Philippines. Ennew uses her exploration of power to explain the dynamics behind the sexual exploitation of children. This is a framework that can be utilised to cast light on our contemporary understandings of child sexual exploitation.

The work of Ennew should be recognised as pioneering – in the United Kingdom policy arena the idea of linking sexual abuse with exploitation did not emerge until around 2005. Before this both the official guidance and practitioners alike tended to use the inaccurate and stigmatising term 'child prostitution' to label what we would now call CSE. This was profoundly unhelpful in many ways. First, it labelled children as somehow being active participants in 'prostitution', which was perceived as bringing the children material gains. Secondly, the male exploiters were constructed as being 'pimps' or 'punters' – rather than being seen as criminal perpetrators. Finally, this 'prostitution' lens for looking at the issue tended to criminalise young people for minor misdemeanours, often relating to offences committed in the process of resisting their exploitation. An example of this way of thinking can be provided from the official guidance issued by the British Department of Health in 2000, where children are clearly criminalised:

> If the child, whether male or female, admits the offence and there is sufficient evidence under s.65 (1)(a) and (b), then a reprimand or final warning should be considered, in accordance with Home Office guidance to the police. (Department of Health, 2000: 6.28)

The shift from utilising 'child prostitution' towards 'child sexual exploitation' is highly significant: we can explore this issue to reflect on the role of theory, research and concepts in helping to shape our modern, contemporary practice. This shift from one concept to the other is summarised in Table 7.1.

Table 7.1 Contrasting perspectives on 'child prostitution' and 'child sexual exploitation'

	Child prostitution	Child sexual exploitation
Perceptions of children and young people	Active role in selling sex for reward	Subject to abuse by perpetrators
Perceptions of involved adults	Pimps and punters	Criminals
Policy responses	Blame and label the children	Prevent, disrupt and prosecute perpetrators
Practice responses	Limited third sector projects, statutory sector punitive or absent	Comprehensive prevention, disruption, prosecution approaches
Media constructions	Child as active, guilty participant	Child as victim of evil perpetrators and failing practitioners

In Table 7.1 we can see that re-conceptualising 'child prostitution' as 'child sexual exploitation' is potentially transformative in terms of policy, practice and social responses. This shows how important our use of concepts and forms of wording are: using the term child prostitution led to some agency responses which were not child-centred and spoke of 'blame' and 'lifestyle choices'. Using the term child sexual exploitation, in contrast, has led to a better understanding of and, therefore, a better response to, this most challenging of social problems.

Reflection point

It has been argued here that the shift from 'child prostitution' to 'child sexual exploitation' has helped to transform policy and practice. Can you think of any other areas of your profession where the language is unhelpful or stigmatising? How could this be changed?

We can also note here that the Jay report (Jay, 2014) into events in Rotherham in South Yorkshire fails to fully understand and utilise this issue of conceptualisation which, it can be argued, undermines the analysis made by Jay of professional understanding and responses in the Rotherham context. The shift from child prostitution to CSE provides a more helpful explanatory framework than the 'blame culture' that emerged in the aftermath of the Jay report and which, in turn, destroyed many otherwise exemplary careers.

It should also be noted, and this is applicable in other contexts, that when politicians and the media call for more 'common sense' from practitioners this absolutely does not work. Common sense would be no guide, whatsoever, in dealing with perpetrators of multiple sexual assaults on children, whose actions often defy any form of common sense. We need well-researched and clearly theorised approaches if we are to effectively safeguard young people: so that we can expect and prepare for the unexpected.

Child sexual exploitation in crisis

The period from approximately 2010 until 2015 saw a major change in understandings of CSE, contrasting to the 'child prostitution' framework explained above, and this shift led to an increase in successful interventions and ultimately in successful prosecutions of groups of perpetrators. These prosecutions led to large-scale media coverage, television programmes and the publication of first-hand accounts by survivors (see, for example, *Girl A: My Story*, by Girl A, for an account of events in Rochdale and *Prey* by Cassie Pike for a remarkably similar outline of events in Halifax).

The state of current understanding is outlined below. In 2017 the English government guidance argued that we need to place CSE in the wider context of child sexual abuse (CSA):

> Child sexual exploitation is a form of child sexual abuse. Sexual abuse may involve physical contact, including assault by penetration (for example, rape or oral sex) or non-penetrative acts such as masturbation, kissing, rubbing and touching outside clothing. It may include non-contact activities, such as involving children in the production of sexual images, forcing children to look at sexual images or watch sexual activities, encouraging children to behave in sexually inappropriate ways or grooming a child in preparation for abuse (including via the internet). (DfE, 2017: 5)

We can then see and understand CSE as a specific form of CSA:

> Child sexual exploitation is a form of child sexual abuse. It occurs where an individual or group takes advantage of an imbalance of power to coerce, manipulate or deceive a child or young person under the age of 18 into sexual activity (a) in exchange for something the victim needs or wants, and/or (b) for the financial advantage or increased status of the perpetrator or facilitator. The victim may have been sexually exploited even if the sexual activity appears consensual. Child sexual exploitation does not always involve physical contact; it can also occur through the use of technology. (DfE, 2017: 5)

In contrast to the Department for Education version, a working definition utilised by the Office of the Children's Commissioner (OCC) is perhaps more graphic and explores the roles of gangs and networks, and the use of threats as coercion, a key feature of CSE:

> Many vulnerable children and young people are caught up in harmful, controlling relationships in gangs where they can be 'traded' as 'goods' or subjected to degrading sexual or unsafe acts amongst its members. Others are sought out by individuals or a group of associates intent on manipulating and sexually harming their victims. Children can remain in these situations for years, unable to extricate themselves because they are confused, afraid or fear reprisals. (OCC, 2011)

It could then be argued that the real impact and nature of CSE, including the brutal nature of the assaults, and the organized nature of the subsequent threats which are often carried out to keep young people in the abuse network, are more exactly outlined in this OCC definition. As mentioned earlier, the nature of CSE is also graphically illustrated in non-academic, but very useful books, such as the one written by the Rochdale victim, Girl A (2013). This book provides a child's view of the experience of CSE and how the grooming process works in detail: it is simultaneously moving, disturbing and informative.

Thus far we have discussed how we can best conceptualise CSE: and that its recent re-conceptualisation established that CSE is a crime with both perpetrators and victims. This is an important shift from the days of 'child prostitution' and 'victim-blaming'. In the aftermath of Rotherham, and other widely publicised cases, the British government is keen to establish that:

> **Child sexual exploitation is never the victim's fault, even if there is some form of exchange:** all children and young people under the age of 18 have a right to be safe and should be protected from harm. (DfE, 2017: 6, bold in the original)

It follows from this that it is important to do away with the language of 'choice', 'consent', 'agreement' and so on:

> Even where a young person is old enough to legally consent to sexual activity, the law states that consent is only valid where they make a choice and have the freedom and capacity to make that choice. If a child feels they have no other meaningful choice, are under the influence of harmful substances or fearful of what might happen if they don't comply (all of which are common features in cases of child sexual exploitation) consent cannot legally be given whatever the age of the child. (DfE, 2017: 6)

The act of 'exchange', it is argued, is central to CSE and is the key that distinguishes it from CSA, a sophisticated argument made by Sophie Hallett in her book *Making Sense of Child Sexual Exploitation: Exchange, Abuse and Young People* (2017). According to the official guidance:

> Whilst there can be gifts or treats involved in other forms of sexual abuse (e.g. a father who sexually abuses but also buys the child toys) it is most likely referred to as child sexual exploitation if the 'exchange', as the core dynamic at play, results in financial gain for or enhanced status of, the perpetrator. Where the gain is only for the perpetrator/facilitator, there is most likely a financial gain (money, discharge of a debt or free/discounted goods or services) or increased status as a result of the abuse. If sexual gratification, or exercise of power and control, is the only gain for the perpetrator (and there is no gain for the child/young person) this would not normally constitute child sexual exploitation, but should be responded to as a different form of child sexual abuse. (DfE, 2017: 6)

We should note that the victims can be male or female, although official statistics suggest that about 80 per cent of victims of CSE are female, and they can be from any ethnicity or social group. Whilst the perpetrator will normally be an older male, peer-on-peer abuse and abuse by females also occur. Often peer abusers may simultaneously be victims – again a situation graphically explored in the book, already mentioned, by Girl A in relation to Rochdale.

Working together to challenge child sexual exploitation

A comprehensive, child-centred and strategic approach to opposing CSE requires, crucially, an effective form of multi-professional practice: building a 'team around the child' is vital to the field of CSE. This connected and coherent approach is discussed by Ofsted, the inspection body, in their publication entitled *Time to Listen* (2016), which found that a coordinated approach is vital:

> some children had too many practitioners involved with them and a lack of co-ordination, together with assessments that did not consider all of the child's needs, meant that support for children was not meaningful to them. (Ofsted, 2016: 3)

This coordinated approach is supported by a young person who stated that:

> I'm sick of telling my story to the YOT worker, the drugs worker, the sexual health worker, the social worker, you, the Connexions worker. (Ofsted, 2016: 3)

It is crucial therefore, and child-centred, that practitioners communicate and coop-erate, a process often enhanced by co-location of practitioners, an issue explored when we discuss the leadership role later in this chapter.

Table 7.2 illustrates some of the professional roles and how a range of practitioners can form a full, comprehensive approach to CSE.

Table 7.2 Professional roles in relation to child sexual exploitation

Professional	Potential primary roles
Social worker	Assessment
	Working with children in need, children at risk of significant harm and looked-after children
Youth worker	Prevention
	Outreach
	Support work
	Group work
Police	Disruption
	Detection
	Prosecution
	Support work
Health visitors and school nurses	Health and development assessment
	Physical, mental and sexual health advice
	Support through pregnancy
GPs and paediatricians	Medical assessment
	Health advice
	Support through pregnancy
Therapists, counsellors, addiction workers	Therapeutic support
	Trauma-informed interventions
Licensing workers	Regulation of licensed premises
	Training taxi drivers, hotel staff, etc.
	Enforcement of licences
Voluntary sector	Preventive campaigns
	Outreach
	Support work
	Group work
	Support for parents (provided by Pace – Parents Against Child Exploitation)

It should be noted that these roles should be both fluid and flexible and practitioners should respond to the specific needs of each young person's situation. The important point is that what is required is to develop a continuum of services that meets the complex needs of young people who are experiencing, or have experienced, CSE.

Reflection point

Using the skill of empathy (discussed in Chapter 9 of this book) put yourself in the shoes of a CSE victim – such as Girl A or Cassie whose experiences were discussed earlier.

What should your professional role contribute to supporting them? How is your professional role distinct from others?

How should you work with other practitioners?

We can summarise the research literature using a publication by Public Health England, which argues that an effective response to CSE is one that:

- is collaborative and multi-agency, with clear roles and responsibilities and clear lines of communication and accountability within this;
- takes learning from the national context but is locally informed and based on an up-to-date understanding of the local profile;
- is contextual, both in terms of locating CSE within a wider context of risk and harm and moving beyond a case by case response;
- straddles both the preventative and responsive agendas; and
- focuses on both victims and perpetrators. (Public Health England, 2019: 24)

The prevention of child sexual exploitation

As with most social and health problems, prevention should be the cornerstone of all professional activity. Prevention in the field of CSE takes us to the core of what we understand to be healthy, loving and respectful relations: schools have a central role here. If young people are supported in those aspects of their lives, then vulnerability to CSE will be minimised.

Practitioners should aim to work universally with young people to ensure they are aware of:

- what a loving relationship looks and feels like
- how to treat a partner respectfully and well
- how to recognise the signs if things are starting to go wrong or are abusive.

There are many resources in the field of personal and social education which can be utilised to develop programmes in this field. Others more directly address CSE – Mr Shapeshifter, for example (see Useful websites, p. 183 for further information).

Whilst such prevention programmes should be universal and school-based there are also more targeted interventions available which can be aimed at specific age groups, or those regarded as 'vulnerable'. An exploration of YouTube will reveal respected videos such as *Chelsea's Choice* and NHS training materials which graphically illustrate the origins and impact of CSE for young people. Practitioners may be able to utilise these in settings such as in-care groups, targeted support groups or residential settings.

There can be little doubt that important developments have taken place in relation to prevention, but there is a significant counter-force which is probably more powerful than all our prevention programmes – that counter-force being the availability of internet-based pornography. Surveys illustrate that almost 100 per cent of teenage young men have utilised such pornography (see www.lancaster.ac.UK/fass/doc_library/edres/12seminars/limmer211112, accessed 16 February 2020) – perhaps giving young men the impression that it is in some way acceptable to dominate and humiliate young women. A social prevention, public health-based programme needs to address this issue and find new ways of promoting healthy relationships, in an extremely challenging wider social context.

This social context is reflected upon by one young woman who was a respondent in Beckett et al.'s study:

> I'm used to it … it's normal … it's wrong, but you get used to it … Welcome to our generation. (2013: 3)

According to this research, young people may have come to take for granted the existence of sexual exploitation, as an inevitable feature of modern life: a sobering thought indeed.

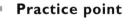

Practice point

How can your professional role contribute to the prevention of child sexual exploitation?

Assessment and child sexual exploitation

Children's social care workers will often be the lead professional in relation to assessment where young people have experienced, or may be vulnerable to, CSE, but it will require effective multi-professional cooperation to develop comprehensive and accurate assessments. It is important to note that we should avoid over-reliance on a checklist/tick-box type approach and that the existence of CSE will involve piecing together a complex jigsaw of factors: in the UK the Chief Social Worker, Isobel Trowler, warned against a tick-box approach to assessment.

The Official guidance identifies the following issues as 'vulnerabilities' which make some young people 'more susceptible to child sexual exploitation':

- Having a prior experience of neglect, physical and/or sexual abuse;
- Lack of a safe/stable home environment, now or in the past (domestic violence or parental substance misuse, mental health issues or criminality, for example);
- Recent bereavement or loss;
- Social isolation or social difficulties;
- Absence of a safe environment to explore sexuality;
- Economic vulnerability;
- Homelessness or insecure accommodation status;
- Connections with other children and young people who are being sexually exploited;
- Family members or other connections involved in adult sex work;
- Having a physical or learning disability;
- Being in care (particularly those in residential care and those with interrupted care histories); and
- Sexual identity. (DfE, 2017: 8)

It is important to note that all young people are potentially victims, and also there is a danger that a focus on childhood vulnerabilities can shift our gaze away from the perpetrators who are ultimately responsible for CSE. No child would be vulnerable if perpetrators did not exist.

There are many potential indicators in a young person's life that may alert us to the possibility that a young person may be experiencing sexual exploitation. Such factors include:

- Going missing from home or care
- Changes in behaviour/sexualised behaviour
- Unexplained gifts/cash
- A new mobile phone, which may be used secretly
- Injuries/marks on the body
- Alienation from a 'same age' peer group
- Increasing secrecy
- Returning home under the influence of drugs/alcohol.

And at the 'heavier end' and, more obviously, in relation to CSE there may be:

- Sexually transmitted infections
- Pregnancy.

There are many practice tools which enable you to achieve a comprehensive assessment. The tool used in Bradford, for example, allows the practitioner to classify a young person as no risk, low risk, medium risk or high risk (see www.bradford.gov. UK/children-young-people-and-families/get-advice-and-support/child-sexual-exploitation/, accessed 16 February 2020).

Whilst such tools can be helpful, it is important to see the young person holistically – they will have strengths and interests, for example, which are important to them. Young people should never be constructed just as a 'problem' or seen simply as 'vulnerable'. Any indicators of vulnerability need to be seen in the wider context of a young person's strengths. Wherever you are working, your own local Safeguarding Children Partnership will have risk assessment forms that you should ensure you are familiar with. Many areas have a multi-agency, co-located team, perhaps based in a 'Hub', where potential CSE situations can be discussed and if appropriate assessed.

Intervention to oppose child sexual exploitation

Once an assessment has been undertaken and the young person may be regarded as a 'child in need', under Section 17 of the Children Act 1989, or if they are seen to be at risk under Section 47, there should be a clear multi-agency plan in place to support the young person, and protect them from CSE. If the young person has been abused, or is looked after within the care system, then the social worker and care staff will have the usual statutory framework in place (medical assessments, reviews and so on) in addition to having a focus on CSE.

A looked-after child who has been subject to CSE will require a care plan that addresses the particular aspects of their abuse. For example, it could be decided to limit the use of the web and/or mobile phones as this will probably be the method used to groom them, and this can continue even when they are placed in care settings. Furthermore, whereas normally with looked-after children a local placement is generally required in the best interests of the child, in the case of CSE, a more distant placement may be required to allow the young person to escape the local network, and/or move away from threats.

Particular support will be required where there are care proceedings or where the perpetrator is being prosecuted. Any court appearance to give evidence requires careful planning and support.

Therapeutic responses

Whereas we have some preventive programmes in place and intervention has no doubt improved since the publication of the Jay report, there is an undeniable and major shortfall in therapy for CSE survivors, a situation which is even worse in regard to perpetrators.

Again this therapeutic and support role is multi-disciplinary and can involve youth workers, social workers, counsellors, psychologists and psycho-therapists (Allnock and Hynes, 2012). As argued in *What's Going on to Safeguard Children and Young People from Sexual Exploitation?* (2011):

> voluntary sector specialist projects are more able to adopt the flexible therapeutic model to which this group of young people is most likely to respond well. This is contrary to the short-term nature of many social care interventions. (Jago et al., 2011: 36)

The therapeutic requirements of young people who have experienced CSE may well be considerable. If you think about someone you know who has been sexually abused by one perpetrator you will know the damage this can cause: imagine if there are five, ten or even thirty perpetrators. In addition, some young women may have a child to one of their perpetrators, and therefore may experience an ambivalent attachment relationship with that child, which they will also require support to address (Frost, 2019).

Understanding ethnicity and child sexual exploitation

It has been argued that:

> child sexual exploitation knows no boundaries. Any child, regardless of where they live, their cultural, ethnic and religious background, their sexuality or gender identity, can become a victim. (Fox, 2016: 2)

Whilst, as the above quote suggests, any child may be a victim of CSE and a person from any ethnic background may be a perpetrator, the Jay report (2014) argued that one reason that CSE remained a hidden and unspoken problem was that practitioners were afraid to speak out about ethnicity in an atmosphere of 'political correctness'. According to Jay:

> there was a widespread perception that messages conveyed by some senior people in the Council and also the Police, were to 'downplay' the ethnic dimensions of CSE. (Jay, 2014: 91)

This is a complex issue to reflect upon and it should be noted that the 2017 Department for Education guidance avoids the issue of ethnicity – apart from saying that perpetrators and victims can come from any community.

It is important to recognise that all children may be vulnerable to CSE and that perpetrators can come from any profession, religion, ethnicity or social class. We know, for example, that many religious settings have been subject to inquiries following widespread allegations of abuse (see www.iicsa.org). Child sexual abuse cannot be assigned to any particular religious background. For example, as discussed in Chapter 4, the English entertainer Jimmy Savile was a committed Roman Catholic – but no one referred to his actions as 'Catholic abuse'.

It remains the case, however, that most of the groups of perpetrators who have been imprisoned for CSE – on-street, group-based grooming of children and young people – have been of Asian heritage and largely Muslim by upbringing (see the Rochdale, Oxford, Bradford and Rotherham cases, for example). Why should this be the case? It would be a dereliction of professional ethics not to explore this issue, when the empirical evidence is so clear.

The connection between CSE and ethnicity may be found in the involvement of men from, for example, Pakistani heritage backgrounds working in the night-time economy. Taxis and take-away restaurants feature in a high-profile manner in first-hand accounts (see 'Child A' and accounts of the court cases). This provides the atmosphere and environment for CSE grooming – under cover of the night, with transport, take-away food and a cash-economy providing an environment in which CSE can flourish. This may well explain the link between ethnicity and CSE, just as the Church or the internet provide environments under which different forms of abuse could flourish.

Whilst all ethnicities contain child abusers and all children can potentially be victims, the link between 'on-street' CSE grooming and ethnicity has implications for practice. Progressive mosques, Muslim women's groups and other Muslim organisations have owned the challenge of CSE perpetrators existing in their community and campaigned against CSE.

Leadership approaches to opposing child sexual exploitation

Given that tackling CSE is ultimately a multi-agency, multi-professional challenge, or requiring what is sometimes referred to as a 'whole systems' or public health approach, it follows that effective leadership and coordination is absolutely essential. Whilst multi-agency approaches require high quality grassroots cooperation, the initial lead and resources need to come from the local leadership, working in the context of national policy.

First of all, leaders need to recognise the scale and importance of CSE – this was perhaps not the case 'pre-Rotherham', but it is certainly the case as this book is being written: however, recognition in itself is necessary but not sufficient.

Second, we require sound multi-agency policies, led by the local Safeguarding Children Partnership. This needs to have support from all the professions, as made clear in the official guidance (*Working Together to Safeguard Children*, HMG, 2018).

Third, such an approach needs to be well-resourced, whether the agreed policy is to establish a co-located 'hub' (see Hill, 2016) or a more 'virtual' resource. It will always be the case that training, agreed protocols and staff resources will be required (Frost and Robinson, 2016).

Fourth, staff will require support and supervision to work in such a demanding field. In multi-disciplinary hubs, careful consideration needs to be given to how this is to work across multi-agency boundaries and address complex issues such as information sharing.

Fifth, and finally, policy and procedure require regular evaluation and review. The nature of CSE, and the technology used to facilitate it, evolves quickly, meaning agencies have to be 'nimble on their feet' in responding to new challenges.

Conclusion

The purpose of this chapter has been to:

- Explain and analyse the impact of child sexual exploitation
- Assess what we understand by the term 'contextual safeguarding'
- Reflect on the changing nature of safeguarding policy and practice.

There has clearly been significant professional learning that took place in the shift from the use of the term 'child prostitution' to the understanding and response to child sexual exploitation. Between 2015 and the time of writing this book this learning has continued and developed through the utilisation of the term 'contextual exploitation', which is becoming increasingly dominant in the field. The meaning and use of this term are explored in the following chapter.

Recommended reading

Sophie Hallett, *Making Sense of Child Sexual Exploitation* (2017)

Drawing on a PhD study this book provides a critical analysis of child sexual exploitation. The author has spoken to young people and practitioners and uses social theory to reach well-argued and clearly evidenced conclusions. This book is highly recommended.

Girl A, *Girl A: My Story. The Truth about the Rochdale Sex Ring by the Victim Who Stopped Them* (2013) and Cassie Pike, *Prey: My Fight to Survive the Halifax Grooming Gang* (2019)

Two first-hand accounts by young women who have survived child sexual exploitation. Well worth reading for the young person's point of view: the two books also contain remarkable similarities.

8

CONTEXTUAL SAFEGUARDING: A CONTEMPORARY CHALLENGE

CONTENTS

The aims of this chapter are to:

- Explore the emergence of contextual safeguarding
- Contrast the implications of contextual safeguarding with traditional approaches
- Analyse recent developments in contextual safeguarding
- Examine the role of the professional in providing contextual safeguarding

Introduction

The period from approximately 2006 until 2015 was highly significant for child safeguarding practitioners and their leaders – it was a period where significant learning took place in relation to the understanding of child sexual exploitation (CSE). There was a shift in focus from exploring events within the household to having a wider view of the context young people live in – thus the emergence of the phrase 'contextual safeguarding'. Contextual safeguarding involves a range of safeguarding challenges including modern slavery, child criminal exploitation, so-called 'county lines' (see Chapter 8), online grooming and radicalisation. Even to list these is artificial as they link and overlap in many ways: they all require a shift towards a contextual safeguarding approach. This chapter outlines the shift towards contextual safeguarding and explores the implications for safeguarding systems, leadership and for individual practitioners.

From child sexual exploitation to contextual safeguarding

As we have argued, there was clearly significant professional learning that took place between the use of the term 'child prostitution' to the understanding and response to child sexual exploitation: this shift took place roughly between 2006 and 2015. From 2015 to the time of writing this book (2020) this learning has continued and developed through the utilisation of the term 'contextual safe-guarding', which is becoming an increasingly dominant approach in the child welfare field. These developments have been led largely by researchers at the University of Bedfordshire (see www.beds.ac.UK/research-ref/areas/social-policy-and-social-work/research-into-child-sexual-exploitation) whose work has significantly influenced government policy and professional approaches. The term contextual safeguarding appeared in the official guidance *Working Together to Safeguard Children* for the first time in 2018, which included the following definition of contextual safeguarding:

> As well as threats to the welfare of children from within their families, children may be vulnerable to abuse or exploitation from outside their families. These extra-familial threats might arise at school and other educational establishments, from within peer groups, or more widely from within the wider community and/or online. These threats can take a variety of different forms and children can be vulnerable to multiple threats, including: exploitation by criminal gangs and organised crime groups such as county lines; trafficking, online abuse; sexual exploitation and the influences of extremism leading to radicalisation. (HMG, 2018: 1:33)

We can see, then, that contextual safeguarding is an approach to understanding and reacting to young people's experiences of exploitation and abuse situated within the wider community. The focus of safeguarding thus shifts from the traditional focus on family and household towards locality and community. By taking this stance practitioners can begin to recognise that young people may face violence, abuse and exploitation in a range of setting situated within the locality or more widely.

One highly significantly issue about abuse in these settings is that it comes between parents/carers and their children; part of the grooming process is to undermine parent–child relations. As argued by the organisation Parents Against Child Exploitation (Pace), parents can feel unable to overcome the very powerful forces within the locality which come between parents and the young person:

> A calculated strategy of grooming, intimidation and coercion by the perpetrators strips parents of their ability to fulfil their parental responsibility. The perpetrators of child exploitation deliberately seek to drive a wedge between the child and their family. (Pace, 2019: 4)

This contextual perspective then potentially changes both the understanding by, and the practice of, child welfare practitioners. It potentially changes assessment practice, skill sets, ideas of prevention, interventions and support processes. Contextual safeguarding, for example, involves attempting to make public spaces safe and may involve mobilising both public agencies and community groups to ensure that this is the case. By using the term contextual safeguarding this in turn changes the aims and objectives of the child protection system by recognising that young people are subject to a range of exploitation in a variety of social and geographical contexts. These issues can only be addressed by effective multi-professional working.

━━━━━━━━ **Practice point** ━━━━━━━━

Check if your agency has a policy on 'contextual safeguarding'.

Make sure you are familiar with the policy.

Do you know who to contact in your agency if you need to know more about the issues raised in this chapter?

Assessment practice for contextual safeguarding

As we have argued above, there are many implications when we begin to think seriously about contextual safeguarding: it requires a significant shift in professional thinking if we are to take into account contextual approaches. This shift includes assessment practice that should take account of the wider context and develop new ways of thinking and acting:

> Assessments of children in such cases should consider whether wider environmental factors are present in a child's life and are a threat to their safety and/or welfare. Children who may be alleged perpetrators should also be assessed to understand the impact of contextual issues on their safety and welfare. Interventions should focus on addressing these wider environmental factors, which are likely to be a threat to the safety and welfare of a number of different children who may or may not be known to local authority children's social care. Assessments of children in such cases should consider the individual needs and vulnerabilities of each child. (HMG, 2018: 34)

This implies that the young person should be seen as existing in the context of neighbourhood, school and peer group, as well as the home. New and different assessment methods are suggested by the research unit based at the University of Bedfordshire in the box below.

....

Undertaking contextual safeguarding assessments

Use different assessment methods – surveys, interviews, policy review, peer assessment

- Context weighting – school culture versus peer group
- Identify policy gaps and staff training needs
- Identify guardians and place managers
- Cultures of harm – normalisation, education needs

- Need multi-agency partners to assess harm
- Can form the basis of traditional Children and Family assessments

This is a shift in assessment practice away from a focus on the household towards the wider community and context: this has profound implications for assessment practice and the lens utilised by practitioners. This Bedfordshire work, and the work of Michelle Lefevre and colleagues (2019), alongside the dissemination work of the organisation Research in Practice, have made the case for a paradigm shift to transform safeguarding work as they argue that:

> There are moral and economic drivers for a re-imagined safeguarding system which is contextual, transitional and relational. (Holmes, 2019)

Theoretical approaches to understanding contextual exploitation

In this section we explore the theoretical implications of working with young people in contextual settings. This work is – to pick up a recurrent theme of this book – both complex and nuanced. For example, it challenges the way we think about 'victims'. Whilst a three-month-old baby who has been abused is clearly a 'victim' and has no agency in this process, this does not apply to young people, who are older, more experienced and have some aspects of agency. They have some qualities of being an agent – they are able to make decisions – and thus in the words of Rees and Stein (1999) make 'imperfect victims'. They are neither simply victims nor straightforwardly responsible for their abuse and exploitation. Sophie Hallett, drawing on interviews with young people and related practitioners, argues how complex and nuanced agency is in relation to CSE:

> If we are to fully apprehend and understand the aetiology of sexual exploitation, young people's agency and more nuanced understandings of risk must be made visible. … This is also a reminder that young people's risky behaviours, and their sexual exploitation, can only be understood in the context of their everyday lives and circumstances – those 'things going on' that can lead a person to feel vulnerable and seek ways to respond to those feelings of vulnerability and powerlessness. (Hallett, 2017: 48)

Along similar lines, Sharland describes young people as being 'agents of their own lives, pursuing their own trajectories, situated within their own social, material, cultural and relational worlds' (2006: 259–60). This argument echoes that of Karl

Marx (1852) that people make history, but not in circumstances of their own choosing. This formulation raises the complex issue of both young people's participation and their protection – and exactly how these two aspects of children's rights work together. One way of addressing this is to build relational, or relationship-based, practice with young people. As part of this perspective the professional 'works with' the young person – as opposed to 'doing to' them: drawing on the principles of restorative practice. The relationship in turn then becomes the vehicle for change rather than safeguarding being something which is imposed or 'done to' the young person. When they are 'done to', young people often report feeling alienated from practitioners and from service provision – they can feel disempowered and disconnected and then this process can in turn increase the risk to them (Lefevre et al., 2019). Even being in a care placement does not always protect the young person – as many SCRs explore (Johnson et al., 2006). In addition, even when they are initially safeguarded, there is a fundamental lack of support for young people who require supportive and therapeutic services, as the current author has argued elsewhere:

> The practitioners (interviewed) value their relationships with the young people, but perceive that there is a lack of specialised, therapeutic services. To address the shortfall will require policy and funding shifts: this is the central challenge for the future of public mental health provision for CSE-experienced young people. (Frost, 2019: 43)

Practice point

Thinking about children and young people you work with, do you know how to access the therapeutic support they require?

Can you play such a role yourself? Can you obtain support in carrying out such a role?

There is a further theoretical issue about the boundary between childhood and adulthood, which relates to the issue of transition. Young people exist across the policy boundary, imposed by practitioners, between childhood and adulthood (Rikala, 2019) – and where as a result a clear divide exists between service structures and policies: a divide which does not reflect the reality of young people's lives and transitions. Support drops when people reach 18, as data gathered as part of an inspection of police services suggested:

> When vulnerable people reach 18, support available to them drops. Interviewees described a 'cliff edge' that is leading to a 'lost generation'. (HMICFRSC, 2020: 4)

Services need to address this issue of transition and ensure that services are more 'joined up'. There are many challenges and shortfalls in effectively providing a comprehensive contextual safeguarding service for young people.

Practice point

When you are working with young people over the age of around 16 try to make sure that they will be supported after their 18th birthday.

For children in care their statutory review should be used to address this issue.

Try to make sure young people are adequately supported once they are over 18.

One way of working towards a more responsive service comes, according to some commentators, from adopting trauma-informed practice (Atwool, 2019). Trauma-informed practice (TIP) is becoming increasingly used to inform professional work in this area, and to address some of the challenges as outlined above. Knight (2019) identifies five principles of trauma-informed practice (TIP) as follows:

- Safety – by which he means keeping the young person safe in terms of relations, physically and emotionally
- Trust – this means building trusting relations and making sure that the young person is not re-traumatised
- Empowerment – Atwool refers here to improving the ability of the young person to make effective decisions that have an impact on their life
- Choice – giving the young person realistic and achievable choices
- Collaboration – here Atwool is referring to working together with relevant practitioners.

TIP practice also embraces the emotional impact of this work on practitioners – within the TIP model they should be fully supported and supervised to help them cope with the difficult circumstances they have faced.

An example of the relevance of trauma-informed practice comes from the experience of unaccompanied asylum seeking children (UASC). This group of children and young people have often experienced trauma – perhaps in a war zone, where often they will have lost members of their family and friendship network.

The UK advisory body NICE suggests the following advice:

Primary prevention will be core to addressing these issues including high quality placements, establishing meaningful and long lasting relationships with adults, establishing friendship networks, culturally relevant networks including those that meet religious, dietary, dress beliefs and needs. Advice and advocacy and links with community networks will also be significant. Contact with or information about family and friends in the country of origin may also be very important. It is essential however, that any of this is driven through consultation and discussion with young people themselves. The resolution of the asylum application will also be very important. Beyond this, the assessment and provision of services for those that are suffering from clinically significant emotional distress and identifiable mental health problems will be important. Accessing CAMH services and other specialist mental health services will be important. But many studies emphasise the need for these services to fully understand the plight and circumstances of unaccompanied minors. (NICE, n.d.: 5)

We can see a direction for future work emerging from the preceding discussion – providing contextual safeguarding which is relationship-based, trauma-informed, addresses transitions and appreciates the rights and agency of young people. These are summarised in the box below.

Towards a young person-centred practice

- Taking account of the wider social context the young person lives in
- Addressing issues of transition in a young person's life – in particular the transition towards adult status
- Building on a relationship-based practice
- Drawing on the principles of trauma-informed practice
- Appreciating the agency of the young person

Reflection point

Think about your current practice or training:

To what degree does this take into account contextual safeguarding?

How can your practice be changed or influenced by the principles of contextual practice: taking into account transitions, relationship-based practice, young people's agency and trauma-based practice?

Elements of contextual safeguarding

Using these ideas we will move on to explore some of the specific challenges of safeguarding children and young people taking into account the wider context of the challenges they may face. This has involved an evolution of the safeguarding mind-set: for example, looking at issues such as modern slavery, which previously would have been seen as existing outside of the narrow remit of safeguarding within the household. Below we explore some of the specific elements of contextual safeguarding – whilst remembering that these distinctions are false in many ways as there is often an overlap between these elements of safeguarding.

Modern slavery

Modern slavery has had a high profile in recent years: where this process involves children and young people under 18, this is a form of exploitation that should generate a contextual safeguarding approach. The International Labour Organization have produced the following definition, as part of their Convention:

> For the purposes of this Convention, the term **the worst forms of child labour** comprises:
>
> a   all forms of slavery or practices similar to slavery, such as the sale and trafficking of children, debt bondage and serfdom and forced or compulsory labour, including forced or compulsory recruitment of children for use in armed conflict;
>
> b   the use, procuring or offering of a child for prostitution, for the production of pornography or for pornographic performances;
>
> c   the use, procuring or offering of a child for illicit activities, in particular for the production and trafficking of drugs as defined in the relevant international treaties;
>
> d   work which, by its nature or the circumstances in which it is carried out, is likely to harm the health, safety or morals of children. (ILO, 1999)

We can see here that forms of contextual safeguarding are connected and that it is artificial to divide modern slavery from child sexual exploitation and 'county lines', both of which are covered by the definition provided above. This is why understandings of different forms of contextual abuse are connected: they all involve the organised exploitation and abuse of power over young people.

Modern slavery will raise many challenges for safeguarding practitioners: young people will be frightened and may be intimidated by gang masters and others who have exploited their labour, and perhaps exploited them sexually too. This form of abuse is difficult for young people to exit from, especially when the threats extend to their wider families. They will require consistent, relationship-based professional support by a multi-professional team. All practitioners, and indeed all citizens, should be aware of the potential signs that someone may be subject to modern slavery.

Possible signs that someone is in slavery

Someone in slavery might:

- appear to be under the control of someone else and reluctant to interact with others;
- not have personal identification on them;
- have few personal belongings, wear the same clothes every day or wear unsuitable clothes for work;
- not be able to move around freely;
- be reluctant to talk to strangers or the authorities;
- appear frightened, withdrawn, or show signs of physical or psychological abuse;
- be dropped off and collected for work always in the same way, especially at unusual times, i.e. very early or late at night.

(Reproduced with the kind permission of Anti-Slavery International. www.antislavery.org, accessed 3 February 2020)

As with all forms of contextual abuse it is possible to disrupt and challenge modern slavery. If you are concerned about a young person potentially being involved in modern slavery you should consult the National Crime Agency website. All known cases should be referred to the National Referral Mechanism (NRM) which collates all known cases across the United Kingdom. The 4Ps strategy is used in relation to modern slavery:

Pursue: prosecute and disrupt individuals and groups responsible for modern slavery.

Prevent: prevent people from engaging in modern slavery.

Protect: strengthen safeguards against modern slavery by protecting vulnerable people from exploitation.

Prepare: reduce the harm caused by modern slavery through improved victim identification and enforcement support

(Local Government Association, 2017)

Modern slavery then is one form of contextual safeguarding, which may not previously have been within the remit of traditional safeguarding practitioners.

Child criminal exploitation and 'county lines'

Another aspect of contextual safeguarding which has emerged in recent years is child criminal exploitation (CCE) and the related phenomenon of 'county lines'. CCE has been defined by the English government as follows:

Child Criminal Exploitation occurs where an individual or group takes advantage of an imbalance of power to coerce, control, manipulate or deceive a child or young person under the age of 18 into any criminal activity (a) in exchange for something the victim needs or wants, and/or (b) for the financial or other advantage of the perpetrator or facilitator and/or (c) through violence or the threat of violence. The victim may have been criminally exploited even if the activity appears consensual. Child Criminal Exploitation does not always involve physical contact; it can also occur through the use of technology. (*Serious Violence Strategy*, Home Office, 2018b: 1)

The attentive reader will note that the wording of this definition shares much with the definition of CSE that we utilised in Chapter 7. Again practitioners and citizens alike should be aware of the potential signs of CCE.

Criminal exploitation of children and vulnerable adults

Some potential indicators of county lines involvement and exploitation are listed below, with those at the top of particular concern:

- persistently going missing from school or home and / or being found out-of-area;
- unexplained acquisition of money, clothes, or mobile phones
- excessive receipt of texts / phone calls and/or having multiple handsets
- relationships with controlling / older individuals or groups
- leaving home / care without explanation
- suspicion of physical assault / unexplained injuries
- parental concerns
- carrying weapons
- significant decline in school results / performance
- gang association or isolation from peers or social networks
- self-harm or significant changes.

(*County Lines Guidance*, Home Office, 2018a)

A specific form of CCE has become known in popular parlance as 'county lines'.

What are 'county lines'?

'County lines' is a term used when drug gangs from big cities expand their operations to smaller towns, often using violence to drive out local dealers and

(Continued)

exploiting children and vulnerable people to sell drugs. These dealers will use dedicated mobile phone lines, known as 'deal lines', to take orders from drug users. Heroin, cocaine and crack cocaine are the most common drugs being supplied and ordered. In most instances, the users or customers will live in a different area to where the dealers and networks are based, so drug runners are needed to transport the drugs and collect payment.

(www.national crime agency.gov.UK)

Again we can see the close connections between CSE, CCE, modern slavery and county lines. The extent of operations such as county lines is difficult to measure but has been assessed as follows:

Current analysis suggests that there are more than 2,000 individual 'deal line' numbers (mobile phone numbers circulated to users to purchase controlled drugs) in the UK, linked to approximately 1,000 county lines. London, Birmingham and Liverpool are the main exporting areas. (HMICFRSC, 2020: 2)

This provides a telling example of the fact that our understanding of child abuse is socially constructed. 'County lines' would have been a mysterious phrase to safeguarding practitioners say in 2010, but has since become part of the everyday media discussion of child exploitation and something that agencies are now having to respond to.

One specific form of 'county lines' has become known as 'cuckooing':

Hundreds of cases of 'cuckooing' have been reported, where heroin and crack cocaine dealers associated with the so-called 'County Lines' supply methodology have taken over the homes of local residents and created outposts to facilitate their supply operations in satellite locations. (Spicer et al., 2019: 1)

Safeguarding practitioners may become aware of 'cuckooing' when they are working with service users who are seen as vulnerable in their communities – care leavers and people with learning difficulties, for example.

It is possible for all the safeguarding agencies to work together to disrupt CCE and other forms of contextual abuse. For example, the Modern Slavery Act 2015 created a number of offences, including 'holding a person in slavery or trafficking for the purposes of exploitation'. It is possible then to prosecute in relation to modern slavery offences against county lines offenders.

There are reported examples of criminals involved in county lines operations being convicted of modern slavery offences as well as drug supply offences. The legislation can make the exploitation of vulnerable people less attractive to criminals. We believe that modern slavery offences should be pursued whenever possible in county lines cases. Some perpetrators may be deterred by the stigma that can come with a modern slavery conviction, particularly involving children. (HMICFRSC, 2020: 31)

Combating CCE requires multi-agency responses, which can be led by the police and/or by the local safeguarding partnership.

Gangs and youth violence

Related to CCE is gang and youth violence, which again can be related to issues such as CSE, and which raises the issue of peer-on-peer violence and exploitation. This is another issue, which whilst it has a long history (see Pearson's excellent study *Hooligan: A History of Respectable Fears*, 1983), has become high profile in recent years with a particular focus on knife crime and the subsequent establishment of Violence Reduction Units by police forces. A gang can be defined as follows:

The word 'gang' means different things in different contexts, the government in their paper 'Safeguarding children and young people who may be affected by gang activity' distinguishes between peer groups, street gangs and organised criminal gangs. (www.nspcc.org.uk/what-is-child-abuse/types-of-abuse/gangs-criminal-exploitation/, accessed 23 February 2020)

These are further defined in the box below.

Types of gang activity

- **Peer group** 'A relatively small and transient social grouping which may or may not describe themselves as a gang depending on the context.'
- **Street gang** 'Groups of young people who see themselves (and are seen by others) as a discernible group for whom crime and violence is integral to the group's identity.'
- **Organised criminal gangs** 'A group of individuals for whom involvement in crime is for personal gain (financial or otherwise). For most crime is their "occupation".'

(NSPCC.org.UK)

The link between gangs and safeguarding young people, as Hanson argues, is as follows:

> Both boys and girls involved in gangs are at heightened risk of sexual exploitation, from others within the gang as well as those outside it. Gangs form a highly conducive context for exploitation for a variety of reasons, including the focus on displaying status and hyper-masculinity through exploitative practices. Childhood neglect is one factor that can create vulnerability to gang involvement, for example via its contribution to youth homelessness and a poor sense of identity, for which gang membership may seem to offer a solution. (Hanson, 2016: 16)

The Office of the Children's Commissioner estimated that in 2018 there were 29,000 children and young people aged between 10 and 17 who were members of a street gang (OCC, 2019). This raises issues about youth culture, about inequality and about the complex transition issue facing contemporary youth. Being in a group or gang is not in itself illegal and not all gangs are criminal. But gang membership may be connected to some of the forms of exploitation discussed earlier in this chapter, including county lines and CCE. The list below, from a US-based organisation, indicates some of the signs that may indicate that a young person is involved in gang activity. Potential signs include that the young person:

- Admits to being part of a gang or 'hanging out' with gang members
- Is committed to certain forms of clothing or logos
- Is particularly interested in gang-based culture – music, websites and so on
- Uses certain gestures to communicate with associates
- Uses gang-based terms and language
- Draws logos and signs on school books, clothes and walls
- Is found to be carrying weapons
- Has unexplained injuries
- Has unexplained cash, gifts or jewellery
- Is often missing from home.

As with other forms of contextual safeguarding, practitioners and citizens alike need to be aware of these factors. Challenging harmful youth gang culture is complex and demanding. The most effective preventive factors rest in universal youth work, which unfortunately has been severely cut during the age of austerity:

> Spending on youth services in England and Wales has been cut by 70% in real terms in less than a decade, with the loss of £1bn of investment resulting in zero funding in some areas, according to research. Analysis by the YMCA youth charity found that local authority expenditure on youth services dropped from £1.4bn in 2010–11 to just under £429m in 2018–19, resulting in the loss of 750 youth centres and more than 4,500 youth workers. (Weale, 2020)

The Child Safeguarding Review Panel, following extensive national analysis, suggests that the following issues should be addressed on a local basis:

- understanding the nature and scale of the problem and identifying children engaged with and at risk from criminal exploitation
- tailored support for front line staff
- service design and practice development
- quality assurance. (2020: 10)

Young people themselves are of course well positioned to speak out on these issues and a group made the following points, specifically in relation to gangs and youth crime, to the British Prime Minister in 2019.

Preventing knife crime

12 points manifesto:

1 Ensuring young people feel safe on the streets is important if they are to stop carrying knives.
2 Work needs to be done to challenge the idea that carrying a knife is the norm.
3 Schools need to provide better support to young people who are at risk of involvement in crime, those excluded from school need a safe place to go.
4 Investment in youth services and mentors is key to helping young people escape violent lifestyles.
5 We need to tackle the underlying causes of violent crime in communities such as lack of housing and unemployment.
6 Gangs need to be prevented from using social media as a means of recruiting vulnerable young people.
7 All media have a responsibility not to perpetuate myths that young people need to carry a knife or contribute towards young people becoming desensitised to violence.
8 Introduce more community police officers who can build relationship and help prevent crime before it starts.
9 Tackling the drugs market is a key part of tackling knife crime.
10 The Government need to provide support to young people who are either already involved or at risk of becoming involved in county lines activity. There needs to be a clear strategy on how to help these victims of exploitation escape involvement with gangs.
11 Custody should be used as a last resort – often it only serves to help young people become 'better criminals'.
12 Rehabilitation, particularly helping young people gain skills and access employment, should be central to the youth justice system.

(Reproduced with the kind permission of All-Party Parliamentary Group on Knife Crime. https://www.barnardos.org.uk/sites/default/files/uploads/APPG%20on%20Knife%20 crime%20-%20Young%20people%27s%20perspective%20August%202019.pdf)

We can, then, prevent youth gang-based violence but this involves investment in young people and adopting the principles of contextual safeguarding. This also involves what is often referred to as a public health approach – looking at prevention, education and community involvement alongside individual interventions. As is argued throughout this book, relationship-based approaches are central. This point is argued in the first national review undertaken by the Child Safeguarding Review Panel:

> Trusted relationships with children are important. We believe that building a trusted relationship between children and practitioners is essential to effective communication and risk management. Establishing such relationships takes time and skill. Above all, persistence, tenacity, creativity and the ability to respond quickly are key qualities required of practitioners. (2020: 8)

Conclusion

The aims of this chapter have been to:

- Explore the emergence of contextual safeguarding
- Contrast the implications of contextual safeguarding with traditional approaches
- Analyse recent developments in contextual safeguarding
- Examine the role of the professional in providing contextual safeguarding.

We have seen in this chapter the emergence of contextual safeguarding as a contemporary safeguarding challenge. The discussion has illustrated the more theoretical points made earlier in the book: that child abuse is socially constructed and that it can change fundamentally over relatively short periods of time. It also illustrates another crucial point: how complex and demanding safeguarding work is: there are no easy answers to any of the issues discussed here. It is also remarkable that many of the issues were not on the professional agenda in, say, 2010. Safeguarding challenges can emerge rapidly and then can change and re-configure just as quickly. It is worth reflecting on what the new safeguarding challenges may be: in another five years, practitioners may be faced with a challenge that we have not even thought of as this book appears in print.

Reflection point

Child sexual exploitation, child criminal exploitation and county lines have all emerged as safeguarding challenges during the first two decades of this century. Practitioners have to be nimble and quick thinking to address these challenges.

Reflect on what you think may be new forms of exploitation that emerge during the next ten years.

Recommended reading

Carlene Firmin, *Abuse between Young People: A Contextual Account* (2017)

Firmin is the originator of the term 'contextual safeguarding' which is now extensively utilised. This book explores the crucial area of peer-on-peer violence and makes a major contribution to our knowledge.

Children's Commissioner for England, 'Keeping kids safe: improving safeguarding responses to gang violence and criminal exploitation' (OCC, 2019)

A comprehensive study of gang violence drawing on a wide range of data and providing some useful and challenging suggestions for improvement.

9

ESSENTIAL SAFEGUARDING SKILLS

CONTENTS

This chapter aims to:

- Explore the skill set required to work with parents and carers in safeguarding situations
- Explore the skill set required to work with children and young people in safeguarding situations
- Promote the skills required in order to maximise participation in safeguarding meetings
- Reflect on the importance of the skills required to chair safeguarding meetings effectively
- Examine report writing as an important underpinning skill
- Reflect upon the use of supervision to underpin effective safeguarding practice
- Explore working with cultural diversity

Introduction

The process of safeguarding children and young people is demanding in terms of emotional labour, the appropriate deployment of skills and the ability to learn and reflect. The challenge of being involved in complex safeguarding practices in a culturally diverse environment – including the home visit, child-centred practice, working with parents and carers and participating in meetings – is explored throughout this chapter. The use of practice support tools will be explored and analysed. This chapter also allows readers to consider these challenging issues and reflect on the personal impact of the work. It is underpinned by the assumption that safeguarding practice is complex and demanding – and therefore requires personal and organisational support. All the professional bodies and associations that are relevant to safeguarding ask members to ensure that their professional skills are kept up-to-date and refreshed so it is important to follow up some of the suggestions for further reading and learning and to take up the multi-professional training that will be provided in your local area.

Practice point

Make sure you are supported in your professional practice. Can you answer the following points positively?

I get regular and high quality supervision

I work in a supportive environment

Senior managers are there for me when I need support

I get regular and up-to-date training

I am aware of agency and multi-agency policies and procedures

I take my annual leave and work a reasonable number of hours each week

If you have responded negatively or you are unsure about any of the above what can you do to improve the situation?

The context of practice

We should all be proud of our particular professional identity. Of course, we face frustrations, barriers and limitations in our roles – but these should not stand in the way of striving to be as good as we can in any role that we undertake. Your sense of professional identity will have been developed throughout your initial training – perhaps the primary role of pre-registration training is to build this strong sense of professional identity. This identity, in many professions, is built through academic and theoretically based input backed up by practice experience – usually called placements. Many of us start as naïve enthusiasts; we develop into novices and then later into our careers become experts – often in a specialist role (a professional development process explored from an adult learning perspective by Michael Eraut, 2012). We also have a personal trajectory (a career) which allows us to change and develop over time. However, this is to over-individualise reality – we all make career decisions, apply for courses and make some good, or perhaps poor, decisions during our lives. But of course, this personal trajectory takes place in a wider social context. Here we consider the role of multi-professional workforce development in providing a context for practice: in reality the individual professional exists and makes decisions by being involved in a complex network of colleagues, processes and procedures.

One crucial role of Local Children Safeguarding Boards (in England they existed between 2005 and 2019) and the subsequent Multi-Agency Safeguarding Arrangements is the provision of multi-agency workforce coordination and development. This is crucial in building a local, effective and connected workforce that offers a high quality safeguarding service. To deliver this requires a workforce development strategy that builds on the specific local situation. By participating in any opportunities that are offered you will develop your own skill set but also contribute to the development of the service in the locality. Developing this skill set perhaps involves two distinct elements: there are 'hard' skills that can be assessed and measured – such as knowledge of legislation, policy and procedures – but also 'soft' skills such as building relationships, team working and communicating. Both skill sets are important in building the fully rounded professional.

========= **Reflection point** =========

Write down issues/skills/sets of knowledge in which you feel comfortable and where you think you are performing well.

1
2
3

Write down issues/skills/sets of knowledge in which you feel uncomfortable and where you think you could be performing better.

1
2
3

Now consult the training and development programme for your local safeguarding partnership/organisation and decide how you can address some of the issues you identified as shortcomings.

We now go on to explore some of the skills required – and how to develop and reflect upon this skill set.

Deploying empathy: An underpinning skill

If there is one essential skill in safeguarding work it is perhaps the ability to deploy empathy and to practise, as a result, in an empathetic manner. Empathy is conceived here as the ability to see any situation through the eyes of another, in everyday parlance to 'walk in someone else's shoes' (Baron-Cohen, 2012). It is useful, for example, to ask before a home visit what will the visit look like through the eyes of a parent or the child?

========= **Practice exercise** =========

You are making a home visit following a referral from a children's centre to a single mother with a four-year-old child. The centre are concerned about bruising on the child's arm.

Using an empathetic perspective:

How would you think that the mother would experience the visit?

How would you think that the child would experience the visit?

What are the implications for your practice?

It is useful to ask the questions in the reflection box above before and after each visit or interaction with a service user. In this case the mother may feel a range of emotions, including being threatened, undermined, angry or even relieved if she feels she requires help. The child may see the worker as a stranger, as much taller than them, they may be frightened to talk in front of mum, or indeed they may open up and start to share their feelings. The range of potential feelings and responses is extensive and after the visit the skilled worker will be able to gauge which factors were in play and why. The important point is that the worker can appreciate the experience through the eyes of the mother or child: this is what we mean by the deployment of empathy. It will contribute to the development of both effective safeguarding and ethical practice.

The home visit

The home visit is central to safeguarding children – it is the crucial practice in many safeguarding cases. It is frequently carried out by social workers – and often by other practitioners, including health visitors, family support workers, school-based staff and police officers. The home visit has been both under-theorised and under-researched in the literature. The work of Harry Ferguson (2011) on the home visit is an important exception, and thus this section draws on, and is inspired by, his work.

The home visit is a central practice for many practitioners who are involved in safeguarding. One key theme of this book is to explore safeguarding as an example of where the State intervenes in the realm of the family: this is one reason why the work is complex and challenging. The threshold of the home – literally and metaphorically – represents the interface between the State and the household.

Whilst the home visit is required by good practice and procedures it is an area that is demanding and often unpredictable. Ferguson describes the home visit as follows, arguing that it:

> requires practitioners to act much more on the basis of knowledge, skill, intuition, ritual and courage than bureaucratic rules and to be craftspeople and improvisers. (2011: 68)

It is also the case that home visiting is deeply a sensory experience: Ferguson's work describes smells, dirt and encounters with threatening dogs, for example. As a consequence he argues that:

> home visiting is shown to be a deeply embodied practice in which all the senses and emotions come into play and movement is central. (2011: 65)

By movement Ferguson is referring to the professional literally moving around the house – from the marginal area of the entrance and the porch, through the sitting room and requesting to see the children's bedroom, as part of an assessment process. The professional in this setting is challenged to improvise and to respond to unexpected circumstances thus using their training, skill set and experience to the full. There are no tick-lists, handbooks or algorithms that can address this complex task: we can, however, provide some points for reflection. Reflective practice is the building block of effective safeguarding.

Before the visit the professional should ask:

What is the purpose of the visit?

What should my approach be?

How will I know if the visit has been successful?

The professional is asked to make many basic, practical decisions in a short period, perhaps including:

Where shall I sit?

Shall I ask for the television to be switched off?

Shall I accept a cup of tea?

In addition, there may be many more challenging professional judgements to make:

Shall I ask to see the child alone?

Shall I ask to see the children's bedroom?

Shall I mention my safeguarding concerns earlier or later in the visit?

In addition to these decisions there are hundreds of micro-decisions to make during a home visit. To fast forward to **the end of the visit the worker may ask:**

When shall I end the visit?

On what note shall I end the visit?

Shall I say when I will visit next?

Practice point

Using the sequence above, reflect on a home visit you have made or are planning and think about:

Before the visit

During the visit

After the visit

and address, as best you can, the questions asked above.

The home visit is deeply symbolic of the power and authority of the State quite literally entering the private realm of the family. Depending on your role you will carry the power and authority of the law. It is argued in this book that the dichotomy between family support and safeguarding is a false one and that any safeguarding function should be offered in partnership with parents, carers and children, wherever possible. Very few parents will be malevolent in their intent – most will have suffered from adverse childhood experiences themselves and research by Bywaters et al. (2016a, 2016b) demonstrates that they are likely to be living in poverty and perhaps in the most deprived areas in the country. Every step should be taken to empower them and improve their lives (see Frost et al., 2015, for practical ideas in relation to this). There is an inherent tension in most home visits between being empowering and 'doing with', sometimes called 'caring', as opposed to being controlling and 'doing to': practitioners are mandated by Section 17 of the Children Act 1989 to do what they can to offer family support, in recognition that for most children the best place for them to be is at home and raised by caring parents.

Working with resistant families

Many families welcome practitioners into their homes, particularly if that help is offered in a restorative and relationship-based manner. Some families, however, may be resistant: this is demanding for practitioners (Shaheed, 2012). This resistance may have a number of causes including:

1   Social disadvantage – the parents may feel that services do not work for them as they may feel they have experienced discrimination in the past.
2   Child protection context – parents may well resist the safeguarding system and fear that their children may be removed.
3   Resisting change – practitioners may be asking for change that the parents do not want to engage with.
4   Denial – the parents may feel that abuse has not occurred and are therefore reluctant to engage with the professional.
5   Professional practice – practitioners need to be restorative, relationship-based and persistent as discussed elsewhere in this chapter (adapted from Shaheed, 2012).

Calderdale Safeguarding Children Partnership provide the following 'Top Tips for overcoming resistance':

- Build a relationship
- Clearly identify the reason for involvement (use plain language)
- Listen carefully to the person's responses; do not jump to conclusions
- Look for positives and strengths in the individual/family/carer's circumstances
- Look forward to solutions, not back to blame
- Maintain trust and be empathic
- Consider the options, make a decision
- Be clear about next steps
- Check understanding. (Calderdale Safeguarding Children Partnership)

The nature of interpersonal communication is crucial to working with resistant families. Whilst most families in the child protection system are poor families, there are examples of practitioners working with neglect in more affluent families. Bernard (2019a) studies this issue and concluded that practitioners:

> have to navigate complex power relationships with parents who are able to use their class privileges to resist their interventions. (2019a: 340)

One of her respondents summarised this as follows:

> Those children are quite hidden, because parents know their rights, they are articulate, and they can be quite avoiding. I would say social workers are quite often concerned working with affluent parents rather than with other parents because they are educated and they are very challenging. (2019a: 343)

Resistance then is complex and hard to work with – but working in these contexts is a core skill that practitioners need to develop.

Report writing skills

An important element of the safeguarding process is report writing. From writing up visits, producing assessments, generating reports in a timely manner for safeguarding meetings and producing reports for the court process, all safeguarding practitioners will spend time, perhaps a considerable amount of time, report writing. It is an important and perhaps under-valued safeguarding skill.

Report writing skills include:

> Writing with clarity. Try not to use unnecessary jargon and explain technical or medical terms.

Write from a strengths-based perspective. Families facing adversity will still have many positives – recognise these in your reports.

Basing your report in evidence – both research evidence and more specific evidence from the actual case. It is important to distinguish between facts and your professional judgement in relation to the situation.

Research with parents and with children and young people consistently shows that they support honesty and transparency. They can cope with bad news if it is fair, evidenced and balanced. Parents will most likely read your report – using our empathy lens mentioned read your report through the eyes of the parents, carers or children. Would they feel it was a fair reflection of the situation?

Safeguarding meetings

As a safeguarding professional you will be involved in a range of meetings including: initial child protection conferences, core group meetings and meetings to consider care proceedings, amongst others. Regardless of the exact nature and content of the meeting the skill set is much the same, and unfortunately is rarely written about in the safeguarding texts. This section explores, sequentially, the skills required in order to conduct yourself professionally at safeguarding meetings. This is a learnt skill and it is beneficial to both service users and other practitioners if we all work to conduct meetings as effectively as possible.

Before the meeting

It is important to plan for a meeting before the meeting commences. You should ensure that you have submitted any required reports, that you are familiar with the details of the case and your role, or potential role, in the case and that you are aware of the logistics (where and when the meeting is to be held). This careful planning will help to ensure that you project yourself in a considered and professional manner at the meeting. Make sure you arrive in good time – being late or searching for a venue at the last minute will not help your presentation at the meeting.

During the meeting

Being involved in a meeting should be an active process – it is part of the 'mutual engagement' we explored earlier – where you are always either contributing or actively listening to the proceedings. Safeguarding is always important: your body language should demonstrate this; you should never come across as being bored or disinterested (or gazing at your mobile phone). When you contribute you should speak confidently and at an appropriate pitch and level for the setting. If you have prepared, as recommended earlier, you should be able to speak with knowledge and a grasp of the facts without constantly consulting your records. You should listen respectfully to all contributions. Your organisation will most probably have an approach to the process – Signs of Safety is often used to enable effective decision making. Many organisations are now committed to restorative or strengths-based approaches. This means that practitioners respect the ability and the strengths that are present in families – these values are exemplified by the process of Family Group Conferences (FGCs). Parents and carers have stated that they appreciate honesty, that they like to be listened to and they like practitioners to deliver what they have promised.

Chairing a meeting

As a student or early career professional you will inevitably participate in safeguarding meetings, and many of you will go on to chair meetings. One career strand is to become an Independent Reviewing Officer (IRO) where chairing meetings is a large part of the working week. Often chairing skills tend to be underplayed in safeguarding texts. The Chair of a child protection meeting will help to establish the atmosphere, the process and the procedure undertaken during the meeting. They will be key to enabling the participation by young people and, where appropriate, their parents or carers. The skill set required by the Chair person is outlined in the box below.

Practice point

The role of the Chairperson – skills and aptitudes

1   Being well organised: you will be prepared, be on time and make sure all the key elements are in place.
2   Being a listener and facilitator: you will understand that listening is an active process and that your role is to enable and facilitate contributions from the meeting participants.
3   Being authoritative: you will carry an air of authority, where people look to you for a steer and guidance. This is very different from being authoritarian.
4   Being a good summariser: you will be able to listen to, absorb, summarise and feedback information in real time.
5   Being a problem solver: you will be able to directly address different perspectives and opinions. You will be able to generate consensus in most situations, and know how to handle conflict when consensus is not reachable.
6   Being a completer: you will be able to reach conclusions, generate action points and check that actions are followed through.

Chairing then is an active process and a skill set that can be improved over time.

After the meeting

Meetings are pointless (you may have been to some!) unless actions are generated and followed through. Many child protection meetings will produce a plan for practitioners to undertake home visits, provide services and undertake monitoring, perhaps through health checks. It is essential that these actions are followed through and recorded and that outcomes are shared on a multi-agency basis. Such follow-up will often take place at Core Meetings (of key practitioners) or at re-convened child protection meetings.

. . . .

What makes effective professional meetings?

Successful multi-agency meetings

What are the expectations of the multi-agency group, parents/carers and the child in the meetings and to achieve desired outcomes? – Is everyone clear about their own role and responsibilities? How is this communicated? Is the purpose of the meeting clear? What will happen if parents do not cooperate with multi-agency meetings and planning? How will members know when there is no longer a need for a multi-agency meeting or plan? What if some members disagree with the decisions made? If anyone identifies any poor practice or is in dispute with any of the other agencies, it is important to use their own agency's 'escalation policy' – this usually means reporting the concern to their own line manager and taking further action as necessary using the multi-agency 'Resolving Professional Disagreements and Escalation' procedure if the matter remains unresolved.

How is the discussion of the meeting structured? – Using a framework will help to maintain focus on the child's needs or risks previously identified. It is important, not just to 'tell the story' but to analyse what that means in terms of impact on the child and progress made to reduce needs or risks. Bringing together single agency chronologies into a multi-agency chronology will assist analysis and provide opportunities to share relevant information.

How is the child's voice/experience taken into account? – The record of the meeting should reflect the child's views about their current and past situation; how their views are being taken into account and influencing the decisions made; how their views and experiences are reflected in the outcome of the decisions made and if not acted upon, why not; how the decision will be communicated to the child. The child's plan should show how the views and daily experience of the child will be obtained.

How is progress assessed? – The child's plan should show clearly how progress is being measured using appropriate tools and measures. The plan should include realistic timescales for the required changes to occur. The record

(Continued)

of the meeting and review of the child's plan should show progress made or lack of it, how this has been measured and by whom.

What if progress is not being made? – All plans should include consideration of a contingency plan which states clearly what will happen if progress is not made within the required timescale. Ideally contingency plans will be discussed and agreed in advance with the child's parents and may include: additional support from extended family members; changes to the child's living arrangements, e.g. temporarily living with extended family, family member leaving the family home; reassessment of risk or need; consultation on statutory action.

When will the plan/purpose of the meeting be reviewed? – This should be agreed and recorded at the first multi-agency meeting.

(Reproduced with the kind permission of the Calderdale Safeguarding Children Partnership. https://safeguarding.calderdale.gov.uk/wp-content/uploads/2019/02/Good-Practice-Guide.pdf)

Working with children and young people

In this book it has been argued that children and young people should be at the centre of the safeguarding process. Featherstone et al. (2014, 2018) have argued that this focus is unhelpful:

> We are … motivated by the concern we feel when we hear the phrase "I'm only here for the child". We understand that the phrase supports the performance of a moral identity in a confusing and frightening landscape where there are multiple vulnerabilities and risks. (Featherstone et al., 2014: 2)

It is argued here that this quote underplays the power differentials between adults and children and therefore also underplays the resultant risk for children and young people. Parton outlines the child-centred approach well:

> This orientation concentrated its focus on the child as an individual with an independent relation to the state. It was not restricted to narrow concerns about harm and abuse; rather the object of concern was the child's overall development and well-being. The programs aimed to go beyond protecting children from risk to promoting children's welfare. (Parton, 2017: 234)

It often emerges from Serious Case Reviews and Child Safeguarding Practice Reviews that the child has indeed not been at the centre of the process. The worker may be distracted by the pressure of their work load, the demands of parents or carers or the overwhelming nature of the family situation. This is one reason that safeguarding work is demanding, complex and can be emotionally draining.

There is a strong body of work that can inform our practice with children – those who have been worked with both in the safeguarding system and those who have gone on to be 'looked-after' in the care system.

In *Working Together to Safeguard Children* the official guidance quotes some (unfortunately unsourced) research about what children want from practitioners.

Practice point

Children have said that they need:

- vigilance: to have adults notice when things are troubling them
- understanding and action: to understand what is happening; to be heard and understood; and to have that understanding acted upon
- stability: to be able to develop an ongoing stable relationship of trust with those helping them
- respect: to be treated with the expectation that they are competent rather than not
- information and engagement: to be informed about and involved in procedures, decisions, concerns and plans
- explanation: to be informed of the outcome of assessments and decisions and reasons when their views have not met with a positive response
- support: to be provided with support in their own right as well as a member of their family
- advocacy: to be provided with advocacy to assist them in putting forward their views
- protection: to be protected against all forms of abuse and discrimination and the right to special protection and help if a refugee.

(HMG, 2018: 1:13)

The message from children and young people then is straightforward and all the messages in the box above can easily be transferred into other forms of practice. There are generic, universal points that apply to all children and young people – treating them with respect, for example. But work with children is also individualised as each child or young person will have their own unique character and experience – grounded in their social class, (dis)ability, gender, ethnicity and other forms of difference. All these factors – which have become known as intersectionality – should be held in mind by the skilful and reflective practitioner.

The practitioner should be aware of the now wide range of tools available on the internet which can give a voice to children who cannot realistically be expected to attend or participate in formal adult-led meetings.

━━━━━━ **Practice point** ━━━━━━

The following website contains free, non-copyrighted material which all practitioners can use to enhance their work with children and give a voice to those children. It is aimed at social workers but can be used by any practitioner.

www.socialworkerstoolbox.com/ (accessed 24 January 2020)

Take some time to explore the website. Take a note of the materials that you may find useful in your direct work with children.

Children and young people from particular social groups – children with English as an additional language and some groups of children with disabilities – will require a particular skill set. For example, the Communication Trust reminds us that communication is about more than just speech:

- Gestures including body language, facial expressions and eye-pointing
- Formal signing systems such as Makaton and British Sign Language
- Symbol support, including paper-based communication tools such as Talking Mats or communication passports and boards
- Written messages
- Voice output communication aids. (The Communication Trust, in Shaw, 2016: 5)

You may not have the required skill set but support and training in communication with children who have specific disabilities will be available in your locality.

The perspectives of children and young people

In an extremely thorough study, Race (2019) explores participation in the child protection process from the perspective of children and young people, social workers, child protection conference chairs and advocates. Race undertook her research with children who had recent experience of the child protection system and utilised semi-structured interviews with children individually or in sibling groups and also undertook focus groups: importantly the researcher used creative, child-centred approaches to enable children to share their views. Race argues that her research:

> found that children want to participate in decisions about their lives and feel that they have much to contribute. However, their experience of participation leads to disappointment and ambivalence. Children feel able to have a say and make their voice heard but are frustrated by experiences of exclusion and inequality and the limitations of their ability to influence outcomes. (2019: 141)

Further she argues that:

> professional intervention serves to enable and facilitate or limit and constrain
> the capability of children to make their contribution in safeguarding processes.
> Whilst professional commitment to child-centred practice and effective
> safeguarding is unequivocal, the discourse of participation is characterised by
> 'yes, but'. At times the focus of practitioners to protect children and to promote
> parental responsibility takes precedence over children's participation. (2019: 141)

Race argues, in a manner consistent with the central arguments of this book, for a reflective and empathetic exploration of participatory practice and that listening:

> to the voices of children enables their contribution to be valued so that children
> can be acknowledged as social actors, able to participate as co-creators of a more
> effective and child-centred safeguarding system. (2019: 142)

Race concludes that children are involved in 'complex power relations' with the adults in their lives and as a result they are involved in an adult-dominated world, which it is difficult for children and young people to influence. The adults, according to Race's findings, tend to place more emphasis on child protection, rather than empowerment and children's rights. Race also points out that:

> the children involved in this research were insightful and able to demonstrate
> their expertise as contributors to child protection processes. (2019: 142)

The power and ability of children to contribute clearly varied in her sample but they all had opinions and experiences that they could share. In Race's sample the majority of children were able to find different ways of being heard and they found ways to participate in safeguarding meetings and also to contribute to decision-making processes. Race argues that the children:

> valued the child-centred, rights-based support offered by advocacy workers and
> the flexibility to contribute in ways that made sense to them. (2019: 143)

The practitioners in Race's sample clearly played a crucial role in safeguarding processes, but for most of the children in her study, their relationships with social workers were difficult to negotiate. Race argues that the urgency of the safeguarding process and the timescale requirements lead to a focus on risk and vulnerability (Parton, 2010). Race's respondents argue that meeting a social worker was overwhelmingly *scary* and anxiety-provoking, as despite the difficulties and tensions within their household, for children the home remained their usual environment and the social workers were intruding upon this. In terms of skills, Race argues that differences in perception, and the unequal power relations, make the development of a relationship of trust between social workers and children difficult, especially in the short term.

Working with children and young people in the safeguarding system

- Bringing empathy and reflexivity to the process of meeting and working with children during safeguarding processes may help social workers to acknowledge their apprehensions.
- Recognising children as participants in the safeguarding process may prompt practitioners to provide them with information about the nature and purpose of the investigation and to negotiate with them about where and how they might work together.
- Working with sensitivity to recognise and build on strengths within the family situation and ensuring their interactions counter rather than reinforce concerns about blame and responsibility for children is important.
- It is evident and commendable that most of the children in this study managed to build more positive working relationships with their social worker over time. This has been found to be integral to positive outcomes for children in safeguarding interventions.
- Interviewees emphasised the importance of being informed about why certain measures were required and what plans were being made. Most of the children in this study did not privilege the importance of the case conference as a decision-making forum. They valued different ways to participate and to make their voice heard.
- In this context it is incumbent upon practitioners to adopt a broad understanding of the safeguarding role, one that recognises the importance of promoting the child's welfare and resilience, well-being and capability in the long term as well as securing their immediate safety.
- From this perspective, there should be opportunities in the safeguarding process for listening and being heard, for the development of self-efficacy and confidence, and for therapeutic approaches that acknowledge the emotional content of the situation.

(Race, 2019)

Race argues against a unilateral understanding of children that sees them as simply recipients of child protection system actions of others. She argues for a conceptual framework which recognises that despite unequal power relations, children and young people are indeed able to exercise agency, at times acting as a protective resource and a change agent, as argued by Linda Gordon (1988). If we see children simply as victims this tends to undermine a strengths-based approach. Race argues for a shift in the culture of child protection that would enhance the experience of children and young people by facilitating their active participation. She expresses some optimism that including creative opportunities in safeguarding processes for children and young people to act as agents will in turn improve decision-making and increase the protective capabilities of children and young people (Race, 2019).

It is useful to conclude this part of the discussion with a quote from one of the young people interviewed by Tracey Race in her study who states that practitioners should:

> have more time with the children, to see how they feel about things and what they think should happen ... It's alright me saying we can fix it, but I don't know how – it's just, I think they should speak to the children more than the adults and make sure children have a say in the decisions. (2019: 143)

Working with parents and carers

Most child protection practice involves working with parents and/or carers (we use the term parent from now on for convenience). It is not possible to generalise their experience: some may be angry, others may be cooperative: some may have harmed their children and yet others will not be responsible for any harm to their children.

Ghaffar, Manby and Race (2012) undertook a study of the experiences of parents and carers in relation to the child protection system. They carried out 42 semi-structured interviews with a total of 47 parents or carers: 39 participants were female and 8 were male. The researchers found that about half of the participants (19) agreed at the time, or with hindsight, that the child protection plan was justified. Approximately the same number (18) felt that the plan had a positive impact on the household situation, mainly as it enabled access to services or provided protection from domestic abuse. Many of the respondents felt that sufficient information had not been provided early on in the process, but that this tended to improve with the passage of time and as relationships with practitioners developed. Unsurprisingly 37 of the 42 households felt that attending case conferences was stressful for them, with five finding attending case conferences a positive experience. The parents were concerned about the number of people attending case conferences and felt that there was sometimes insufficient time to read reports prior to the conference. They were largely positive about the chairing and facilitation of the case conferences. Parents generally found the smaller, more focused, Core Groups to be a more positive experience. Again about half (18) felt positive about the consultation process and that their views were taken into account. Most of the respondents (27) thought that multi-professional communication was good and around three-quarters felt they had a positive relationship with at least one professional. The parents valued straightforwardness, honesty, being child-centred and practical help was appreciated.

A small group (7) felt that they had been stigmatised by the process. Some parents (19) were concerned about how often social workers were changed and that the quality of service varied depending on the social worker they were working with. Twenty-four households reported that they had received an effective package of support. Twenty-five households said that parental mental health was a factor in their lives: but received mixed levels of support in relation to this. Twenty-five of the respondents had experienced domestic abuse, with 6 feeling that they had experienced good levels of support in relation to this. Seventeen households faced financial challenges: but only a minority felt that they had received support in relation to this.

Drawing on this important study and other related work there are some useful practice principles that can be followed in working with parents and carers as follows:

1 All parents should be treated with respect: they should be listened to and information should be shared fully and comprehensively wherever possible.
2 Parents respond well to honesty: whether this is good or not so good news. They value time being spent with them by practitioners. It is worth remembering that if your assessment of the situation is accurate then the parents will know this.
3 It may be possible to work more creatively with a protective parent – who will often be the mother. An alliance may be built with a protective parent to ensure that the child is effectively safeguarded.
4 In cases of contextual safeguarding the parents may feel disempowered and as if they are secondary victims of the situation.

Some parents may seem to be cooperative but may actually not be working alongside the professional: this is sometimes called 'disguised compliance'. The skilled and experienced professional may be able to identify this and provide an appropriate challenge to the parent(s).

A very powerful example of good quality practice comes from the court case known as Re D (A Child) (No. 3) [2016] EWFC 1. Lord Justice Munby describes the letter quoted below as follows:

I commend his powerful words to every family judge, to every local authority and to every family justice professional in this jurisdiction.

The letter was written by a social worker to parents who had learning difficulties and represents high quality safeguarding work – based on the principles of empathy and family support.

Model letter to parents

I am writing to you because I am very worried that you are not able to look after D and give him what he needs. I am so worried about D that I am thinking that he may need to be looked after by other carers. These are my worries:

1   I am worried because I sometimes see D come to you, and you do not respond to him. I am worried that D is not getting the cuddles he needs. I am worried that you do not speak to D enough and you do not give him enough praise.

2   I am worried because D is falling behind in his development. I am worried that you do not help D progress in his development. This is because practitioners have shown you how to play with D and told you how to help D learn to improve his speech, but you do not provide D with enough play and talking to when you are at home.

3   I am worried because I and other practitioners visiting your home have seen D hitting, throwing and shouting. The Family Nurse has helped you to show D that he must not do this. I am worried because you have not been able to provide consistent guidance to D and he does not know that this is wrong. I am worried that D does not understand from you what he is and is not allowed to do.

4   I think you need to think more about D's safety when you are out and about. I am worried that you do not always look after D when you are out and about or in the home, for example, when he was able to get into the road. I am worried that you do not always notice what he is doing in the home, for example, picking up a kitchen knife during a visit from a child social care worker and D jumping on chairs. D could be hurt.

5   I am worried that you have had lots of advice and support from practitioners and my worries for D are still present. I am worried that you are not able to look after him and give him what he needs so that he can reach his full potential.

6   I am also very worried that I have received information that you have taken D to see [his uncle G] without the permission of the Children Services. I have previously shared my concerns with you that D may not be safe with G and have only recently repeated this concern to you.

7   I am worried that D is developmentally delayed and may have additional learning needs and this means he will need lots more care than a parent would normally be expected to provide. Over the past two years, you have both needed a lot of extra support to help you care for D. Even with this support, you have continued to find it hard to give D what he needs so that he is growing as well as he could be.

I want to let you know that I am going to be meeting with someone from our legal team to talk about placing D with other carers. I also want to give you the opportunity to have a think about this letter and tell me how you think you may be able to help me not to be worried about D any more.

This letter is a model of effective safeguarding work, which is simultaneously working together with parents, using transparency and honesty.

Working with cultural diversity

All safeguarding practitioners need to be aware of the cultural diversity they work within. Working in the safeguarding field is emotionally demanding and the challenges may be more demanding where there are ethnic and cultural differences between the professional and the family they are working with. Many communities today are 'super diverse' (Meissner and Vertovec, 2015) containing populations with a wide variety of ethnic backgrounds. This chapter is focused on the skill set required in safeguarding and specifically here in relation to work in culturally diverse settings. The organisation Research in Practice suggest the following principles for culturally confident practice: the messages are consistent with those given elsewhere in this book. The basic principles are as follows:

Being child-centred: a focus on the child and being aware of the development and needs of the child. This can be guided using a tool provided by WHO – www.who.int/childgrowth/en. Cultural concerns should not impede effective safeguarding if the child is at risk.

Relationships at the core: building culturally aware relationships with adults and children alike is crucial. We need to be aware that 'colour blind' ('I treat everyone the same') approaches are not helpful: we need to respond appropriately to the full variety of cultural needs and differences.

Knowledge of risk factors: avoiding cultural stereotypes is important; they will often be misplaced and may mean that the professional is not fully aware of risks.

Parenting styles and physical punishment: there are a wide variety of culturally based parenting practices which should be supported and encouraged as long as they promote the best interests of children and young people. Where this is not the case – for example the excessive use of physical punishment within the household – this should be discouraged and legal sanctions can be utilised if required.

Religion as risk and resilience factor: most faith practices are supportive for children and young people, and faith communities are an important aspect of resilience and support for families.

However, some minority faith beliefs support the use of witchcraft or female genital mutilation, for example (see the Victoria Climbié report, Laming, 2003). Again these should be challenged and legal interventions utilised if required. Local Multi-Agency Safeguarding Partnerships should build effective partnerships with community-based faith groups to develop shared and joint approaches. Some faiths or cultures support female genital mutilation (FGM): this is clearly child abuse and is a criminal offence. All cases of FGM must be reported to the Department of Health and Social Care and in cases of girls under 18 to the police and social care. Support can be obtained from the NSPCC FGM helpline (0800 028 3550) and from progressive women's groups such as NESTAC (New Step for African Community).

Underpinned by reflective practice: as with all safeguarding practice, reflective practice, based in principles of equality and social justice, should underpin work with culturally diverse communities. (Adapted from Bowyer, 2015)

Reflection and supervision

Given the complexities of the home visit, and all the other safeguarding tasks discussed in this book, reflective practice and supervision are essential to ensuring that safeguarding practice is of the highest standard. What is meant by reflection or reflective practice? It is the ability to think about, process and re-process actions that we have taken: in this context we are referring to child safeguarding practice but it could be applied to any sphere of life. We should reflect before an action: for example, why am I undertaking this home visit, what am I trying to achieve and how should I behave to achieve these outcomes? This reflection before the event should help improve the quality of professional practice. During the home visit it is also important to reflect – although this is demanding as the professional has to think 'on their feet'. This reflection is sometimes called 'tacit': that is, something that becomes more intuitive as the professional gains experience. The reflective cycle then enters the post-activity phase: were the outcomes as we anticipated, what went well and what could have gone better and what needs to change and happen next? The reflective process then commences again. In a classic formulation Tony Morrison (1993) saw this as a cycle moving from:

Plan and Act to

Experience to

Reflection to

Analysis

There are many models of reflection: one that is often utilised comes from Graham Gibbs (1988):

Description of the experience

Feelings and thoughts about the experience

Evaluation of the experience, both good and bad

Analysis to make sense of the situation

Conclusion about what you learned and what you could have done differently

Action plan for how you would deal with similar situations in the future, or general changes you might find appropriate.

This reflective cycle is important in all professional spheres: a university lecturer, for example, would no doubt improve their lectures if they followed this process. It is, however, absolutely crucial in the sphere of safeguarding where the best interests and welfare of children and young people are at stake. As the stakes are high and the pressures are often significant, reflection is crucial. For example, a parent may have been angry when the purpose of the visit was explained. The worker can use the space provided by reflection to think about this anger: was it, for example, genuine anger that an injustice had been done, or was the anger rather cover for abusive actions undertaken by the parent? Reflection is, or rather should be, central to the safeguarding process: it is essential to safeguarding children and young people.

Reflection can be a solitary activity: supervision is a more shared and supportive activity where reflection can take place. Supervision provides an environment where views, events and reflections can be shared, discussed and where necessary challenged. This process, when carried out effectively, can improve practice particularly when carried out skilfully and empathetically. Supervision can take a number of forms:

- One-to-one supervision – is usually formal and part of organisational procedures. It should be planned and recorded. This supervision should be undertaken in private and the time and space should be valued and respected.
- Group supervision – can be used to explore case studies, for example when a worker is feeling 'stuck' with a particular case.
- Improvised, or ad hoc, supervision – takes place in the kitchen or over the photocopier, for example, and can be an important support for addressing smaller issues or where an urgent steer is required. It cannot replace formal, one-to-one supervision. The box below summarises the underpinning principles of reflective supervision.

Six principles of reflective supervision

1   To deepen and broaden workers' knowledge and critical analysis skills
2   To enable confident, competent, creative and independent decision-making
3   To help workers build clear plans that seek to enable positive change for children and families
4   To develop a relationship that helps staff feel valued, supported and motivated
5   To support the development of workers' emotional resilience and self-awareness
6   To promote the development of a learning culture within the organisation.

(Earle et al., 2017. Reproduced with the kind permission of Research in Practice, a department of Dartington Hall Trust.)

These are not simply abstract points; they need to be put into practice by practitioners. The box below outlines some useful points for reflection in practice.

Practice point

Before the visit

The worker should reflect on what is the purpose of this visit? What am I expecting to change as the result of the visit? What professional behaviours should I adopt to achieve the results that I want? How should I respond to the unexpected, e.g. a new partner being present, the parent being unexpectedly hostile and so on?

During the visit

The worker should reflect, wherever possible, on the nature of the visit: is it going as expected, how can I change the direction of the visit if required, how shall I summarise the visit on its conclusion?

After the visit

The worker should ask: how did the visit go, what went well and what could have gone better, what needs to happen at the next meeting?
The reflective cycle should then start again.

Conclusion

This chapter has attempted to:

•   Explore the skill set required to work with parents and carers in safeguarding situations

- Explore the skill set required to work with children and young people in safeguarding situations
- Promote the skills required in order to maximise participation in safeguarding meetings
- Reflect on the importance of the skills required to chair safeguarding meetings effectively
- Examine report writing as an important underpinning skill
- Reflect upon the use of supervision to underpin effective safeguarding practice
- Explore working with cultural diversity.

This chapter has acted as an exploration of the skill set required to work in the field of safeguarding children and young people. Each of the topics explored in the chapter could be the subject of a book in itself. Readers are encouraged to consult the items listed in the recommended reading below, and explore the useful websites listed on p. 183–4. Safeguarding, as this book has argued throughout, is complex and very demanding of professional skills and emotional labour: we all have a professional duty to learn and to reflect as we practise.

Recommended reading

Brid Featherstone and colleagues, *Protecting Children: A Social Model* (2018)

A book which argues that much is wrong with the current system. It draws on theory and research, but also provides practical case studies which apply the ideas that are presented in practice.

Harry Ferguson, *Child Protection Practice* (2011)

This book explores practice in a day-to-day setting, through the lens of social theory and drawing on the author's direct observation of practice.

10

CONCLUSION AND LEARNING FOR THE FUTURE

CONTENTS

This chapter will bring together the main learning points from this text and provide a summary of the key learning. The book has attempted to cast some light and coherence on an area that is extensively written about and reflected upon. Safeguarding, as we have seen, is a topic that is controversial and often enters the arena of public and political debate. The book has developed a number of guiding propositions:

1   Our understanding and response to safeguarding is socially constructed. This means that understandings of abuse are constructed by social forces that vary across time and geography. This process shapes practice in specific situations.
2   Safeguarding work should be underpinned by the professional skills and values discussed in the book: the most significant of these is mobilising empathy as a central approach in building relationship-based practice.
3   Safeguarding practice is always complex and demands significant emotional labour.
4   Safeguarding practice and policy are a key marker of the relationship between the State and the household: this is why it is complex, demanding and at times controversial.
5   A blame culture (except in cases of clear professional negligence) is unhelpful in the safeguarding world where the vast majority of practitioners are fully committed and hard-working in addressing complex everyday challenges.
6   Safeguarding practitioners need to be highly educated, well supported and adequately resourced in order to carry out their complex work. In return they need to commit to continuing professional development and keeping abreast of new developments, research, and legal and policy changes.

In the course of the book we hope to have provided a rationale and supporting evidence for (a) – (f) above. The learning has been underpinned by reflection points, practice points and further reading.

A safer world for children and young people?

All safeguarding practitioners want the world to be a safer place for children and young people: that is the purpose of their work each and every day. All practitioners should be dedicated to safeguarding the individual children they work with and should campaign against the underlying causes of child maltreatment whenever they can. We can note optimistically that in some ways the world is becoming safer for children and young people:

1   There is a wider recognition of children's rights and voice backed up by attempts to implement the recognition of these universally through the UNCRC.
2   There are attempts to implement prevention programmes, such as the WHO INSPIRE initiative which is discussed later in this chapter.

3   There are improved intervention programmes in areas such as child sexual exploitation and internet abuse.
4   There is a growth of professional knowledge of safeguarding, as demonstrated throughout this book.

But unfortunately, the world is becoming more dangerous for children and young people, as follows:

1   The widespread availability of pornography on the internet means that young people can be socialised into a world where sexuality is learnt on the internet, in a way often associated with the degradation of women and the easy availability of sexual gratification.
2   The internet provides numerous ways that children can groomed and abused – locally, regionally and internationally.
3   Abusers seem to be able to devise new ways of abusing children and young people – the use of young people in criminal exploitation being an example which has been recognised in recent times.
4   Global social change – brought about by war, conflict and climate change – makes children more mobile, perhaps separated from safer environments and more vulnerable to abuse and exploitation.
5   Poverty and inequality act as breeding grounds for child maltreatment – and these social divisions are increasing in many parts of the world.

It is not possible to say – balancing these complex developments – if the world is becoming a safer place for children, or a more dangerous place. Most likely there is a complex interplay of factors which makes it hard, if not impossible, to reach an informed position on this and what future developments there may be.

Towards a safer world for children and young people

We all have a professional duty towards making the world a safer place for children and young people. We will use the INSPIRE framework to help us here. The points in bold are drawn from the INSPIRE framework.

We should create safe, sustainable and nurturing family environments, and **provide specialised help and support for families at risk of violence**, which is perhaps the main point explored in this book. This involves many ways of working with families, including challenging poverty, inequality and social exclusion. At a household level we need to work with parents and carers to improve family environments for children. It is remarkable that as a society the challenges of being a parent are not fully recognised, with little universal education available.

Being able to **modify unsafe environments through physical changes** is crucial. In countries such as Angola, where children are blown up by landmines, or in Bangladesh, where factory fires and building collapses kill children, environmental issues are central to the safety of children and young people. In the Western world we saw in our analysis of contextual safeguarding that the environment also needs to be more child- and young person-centred.

We need to **reduce risk factors in public spaces (e.g. schools, places where young people gather) to reduce the threat of violence**, which is fundamental, whether it refers to children who may be shot at college in the USA, or young people in the UK, who as we have seen are vulnerable to contextual abuse in many public spaces.

We need to prioritise addressing **gender inequities in relationships, the home, school, the workplace**, which is vital in undermining one of the root causes of the abuse of girls and young women. Throughout this book we have argued that power inequalities lie at the heart of the causation of abuse. As child abuse is fundamentally about the abuse of power, addressing gender inequities is crucial.

Engaging in changing **the cultural attitudes and practices that support the use of violence**, again is vital. Attitudes that see children as 'acceptable' victims, whether at school or in the home, require a fundamental value shift. Children and young people are citizens in their own right and not the property of adults.

By ensuring that **legal frameworks prohibit all forms of violence against children and limit youth access to harmful products, such as alcohol and firearms**, we can reduce child maltreatment as part of the value shift discussed in the point above.

As practitioners we all have a duty to **provide access to quality response services for children affected by violence** and other forms of maltreatment.

We also have a more demanding professional duty to **eliminate the cultural, social and economic inequalities that contribute to violence, close the wealth gap and ensure equitable access to goods, services and opportunities**.

Finally, as has been emphasised throughout this book, we must all do what we can to **coordinate the actions of the multiple sectors that have a role to play in preventing and responding to violence against children.** (INSPIRE, WHO, 2018: 20)

We end with a quote from a leading commentator, Professor Nigel Parton:

the challenges of child protection are now much wider than just focusing upon the relationship between the state and the family and … the sites for the maltreatment and abuse of children and young people are now much wider and include various institutions and the wider community. Attempts to analyse and compare child protections systems need to try and address these challenges. This is particularly the case as there is an increasing recognition that violence against children is a global problem which takes different forms in different places. (Parton, 2017: 239)

GLOSSARY

Adverse childhood experiences A range of negative experiences during childhood which may have adverse consequences during adulthood.

Child abuse Forms of violence and abuse against children and young people which may be active acts of commission, or perhaps inaction, which lead to negative consequences for children.

Child criminal exploitation Where an individual or group takes advantage of an imbalance of power to coerce, control, manipulate or deceive a child or young person under the age of 18 into any criminal activity (a) in exchange for something the victim needs or wants, and/or (b) for the financial or other advantage of the perpetrator or facilitator and/or (c) through violence or the threat of violence. The victim may have been criminally exploited even if the activity appears consensual. Child criminal exploitation does not always involve physical contact; it can also occur through the use of technology (Home Office, 2018b: 1).

Child protection Activities undertaken in response to actual or potential harm to children and young people.

Child sexual abuse May involve physical contact, including assault by penetration (for example, rape or oral sex) or non-penetrative acts such as masturbation, kissing, rubbing and touching outside clothing. It may include non-contact activities, such as involving children in the production of sexual images, forcing children to look at sexual images or watch sexual activities, encouraging children to behave in sexually inappropriate ways or grooming a child in preparation for abuse (including via the internet) (DfE, 2017: 5).

Child sexual exploitation Child sexual exploitation is a form of child sexual abuse. It occurs where an individual or group takes advantage of an imbalance of power to coerce, manipulate or deceive a child or young person under the age of 18 into sexual activity (a) in exchange for something the victim needs or wants, and/or (b) for the financial advantage or increased status of the perpetrator or facilitator. The victim may have been sexually exploited even if the sexual activity appears consensual. Child sexual exploitation does not always involve physical contact; it can also occur through the use of technology (DfE, 2017: 5).

Contextual safeguarding   As well as threats to the welfare of children from within their families, children may be vulnerable to abuse or exploitation from outside their families. These extra-familial threats might arise at school and other educational establishments, from within peer groups, or more widely from within the wider community and/or online. These threats can take a variety of different forms and children can be vulnerable to multiple threats, including: exploitation by criminal gangs and organised crime groups such as county lines; trafficking, online abuse; sexual exploitation and the influences of extremism leading to radicalisation (HMG, 2018: 1:33).

County lines   County lines is a term used when drug gangs from big cities expand their operations to smaller towns, often using violence to drive out local dealers and exploiting children and vulnerable people to sell drugs. These dealers will use dedicated mobile phone lines, known as 'deal lines', to take orders from drug users. Heroin, cocaine and crack cocaine are the most common drugs being supplied and ordered. In most instances, the users or customers will live in a different area to where the dealers and networks are based, so drug runners are needed to transport the drugs and collect payment (National Crime Agency).

Emotional abuse   The persistent emotional maltreatment of a child such as to cause severe and persistent adverse effects on the child's emotional development. It may involve conveying to a child that they are worthless or unloved, inadequate, or valued only insofar as they meet the needs of another person. It may include not giving the child opportunities to express their views, deliberately silencing them or 'making fun' of what they say or how they communicate. It may feature age or developmentally inappropriate expectations being imposed on children. These may include interactions that are beyond a child's developmental capability, as well as overprotection and limitation of exploration and learning, or preventing the child participating in normal social interaction. It may involve seeing or hearing the ill-treatment of another. It may involve serious bullying (including cyber bullying), causing children frequently to feel frightened or in danger, or the exploitation or corruption of children. Some level of emotional abuse is involved in all types of maltreatment of a child, though it may occur alone (HMG, 2018: 104).

Female genital mutilation   Female genital mutilation (FGM), also called 'cutting', involves the removal of some or all of the external parts of a girl's genitalia (World Health Organization).

Modern slavery   A form of exploitation and abuse. The worst forms of child labour, as defined by an ILO Convention, comprise:

a   all forms of slavery or practices similar to slavery, such as the sale and trafficking of children, debt bondage and serfdom and forced or compulsory labour, including forced or compulsory recruitment of children for use in armed conflict;

b   the use, procuring or offering of a child for prostitution, for the production of pornography or for pornographic performances;

c   the use, procuring or offering of a child for illicit activities, in particular for the production and trafficking of drugs as defined in the relevant international treaties;

d   work which, by its nature or the circumstances in which it is carried out, is likely to harm the health, safety or morals of children (ILO, 1999).

Multi-disciplinary working   How a range of practitioners work together across their disciplines and organisational boundaries.

Neglect   The persistent failure to meet a child's basic physical and/or psychological needs, likely to result in the serious impairment of the child's health or development. Neglect may occur during pregnancy as a result of maternal substance abuse. Once a child is born, neglect may involve a parent or carer failing to:

a   provide adequate food, clothing and shelter (including exclusion from home or abandonment)

b   protect a child from physical and emotional harm or danger

c   ensure adequate supervision (including the use of inadequate caregivers)

d   ensure access to appropriate medical care or treatment.

It may also include neglect of, or unresponsiveness to, a child's basic emotional needs (HMG, 2018: 105).

Physical abuse   A form of abuse which may involve hitting, shaking, throwing, poisoning, burning or scalding, drowning, suffocating or otherwise causing physical harm to a child. Physical harm may also be caused when a parent or carer fabricates the symptoms of, or deliberately induces, illness in a child (HMG, 2018: 103).

Safeguarding   Safeguarding children and young people is a wider activity than child protection and includes the prevention and responding to child abuse in all its forms.

Social construction   Is the process by which understanding of phenomena in the social world are shaped by interpretations and perspectives. The same issue may be understood differently depending on the historical and geographic context in which the phenomena occur.

Victim/survivor   Victims become survivors when it becomes clear that the abuse was not their fault and responsibility sits with the perpetrator of the abuse. A victim can become a survivor if they are resilient and when supported by others.

USEFUL WEBSITES

Action for Children

www.actionforchildren.org.uk/

A useful NGO website covering a wide range of issues including safeguarding and a number of campaigning issues.

Barnardo's

www.barnardos.org.uk/

One of the UK's leading NGOs with an extensive website providing excellent coverage of many safeguarding issues. Particularly strong on issues relating to exploitation – Barnardo's is the largest provider of CSE support services in the country.

Centre of Expertise on Child Sexual Abuse

www.csacentre.org.uk

A UK-based organisation bringing together a range of expert partners with a focus on child sexual abuse. The website contains a large number of useful reports.

Independent Inquiry into Child Sexual Abuse

www.iicsa.org.uk

An extensive website providing information on the UK-based Independent Inquiry into Child Sexual Abuse. The inquiry commissions relevant research and has produced a number of reports on the different threads of the inquiry.

Mr Shapeshifter

www.mrshapeshifter.com/

One example, amongst many, of useful and imaginative online sources for working with young people on sexual exploitation issues. This is an animation which raises many crucial issues for children and young people.

NSPCC

www.nspcc.org.uk/

One of the leading safeguarding NGOs in the United Kingdom. An extensive range of campaigning, research and policy information on all aspects of safeguarding.

NWG

www.nwgnetwork.org

A valuable UK-based website providing access to hundreds of reports relating to child sexual exploitation and contextual safeguarding.

Pace

www.paceuk.info

Parents Against Child Exploitation is a UK-based organisation that works with parents. They have co-located staff based with some multi-disciplinary hubs. Their website contains useful information for parents and professionals.

Social workers toolbox

www.socialworkerstoolbox.com/

A treasure trove of materials that can be used by any practitioner for imaginative direct work with children and young people.

UNICEF

www.unicef.org

UNICEF is part of the United Nations and aims to ensure that 'every child has the right to grow up in a safe and inclusive environment'. It 'works with partners around the world to promote policies and expand access to services that protect all children'. This website offers a wide range of research-based reports.

WHO

www.who.int/

The World Health Organization coordinates international health-based initiatives. They provide extensive and well-researched data on many safeguarding issues, taking a global perspective.

REFERENCES

All-Party Parliamentary Group on Knife Crime (2019) *Young people's perspectives on knife crime* available at: https://www.barnardos.org.uk/sites/default/files/uploads/APPG%20on%20Knife%20crime%20-%20Young%20people%27s%20perspective%20August%202019.pdf (accessed 16 June 2020).

Allen, A. and Morton, A. (1961) *This is Your Child: The Story of the National Society for the Prevention of Cruelty to Children.* London: Routledge & Kegan Paul.

Allnock, D. and Hynes, P. (2012) *Therapeutic Services for Sexually Abused Children and Young People: Scoping the Evidence Base.* London: NSPCC.

Ariès, P. (1965) *Centuries of Childhood: A Social History of Family Life.* New York: Vintage.

Ashton, K., Bellis, M. and Hughes, K. (2016) 'Adverse childhood experiences and their association with health-harming behaviours and mental wellbeing in the Welsh adult population: a national cross-sectional survey', *The Lancet, 388*: 21.

Astbury, J. (2013) *Child Sexual Abuse in the General Community and Clergy-Perpetrated Child Sexual Abuse: A Review Paper.* Melbourne: The Australian Psychological Society.

Atwool, N. (2019) 'Challenges of operationalizing trauma-informed practice in child protection services in New Zealand', *Child & Family Social Work, 24*(1): 25–32.

Baginsky, M. and Holmes, D. (2015) *A Review of Current Arrangements for the Operation of Local Safeguarding Children Boards.* London: LGA /RIP.

Baron-Cohen, S. (2012) *The Science of Evil: On Empathy and the Origins of Cruelty.* New York: Basic Books.

Barter, C. (1999) 'Practitioners' experiences and perceptions of investigating allegations of institutional abuse', *Child Abuse Review, 8*(6): 392–404.

Bass, E. and Davis, L. (1988) *The Courage to Heal.* New York: HarperCollins.

Beckett, H., Brodie, I., Factor, F., Melrose, M., Pearce, J., Pitts, J., Shuker, L. and Warrington, C. (2013) '"It's wrong – but you get used to it": a qualitative study of gang-associated sexual violence towards, and exploitation of, young people in England'. Luton: University of Bedfordshire.

Behlmer, G.K. (1982) *Child Abuse and Moral Reform in England, 1870–1908.* Stanford, CA: Stanford University Press.

Bell, V. (2002) *Interrogating Incest: Feminism, Foucault and the Law.* London: Routledge.

Bellfield, C.R., Noves, M. and Barrett, W.S. (2006) *HighScope Perry Pre-school Program: Cost Benefit Analysis using data from the age 40 year follow up.* New Brunswick: NIEER.

Bernard, C. (2019a) 'Recognizing and addressing child neglect in affluent families', *Child & Family Social Work, 24*(2): 340–7.

Bernard, C. (2019b) 'Working with cultural and religious diversity'. In Horwath, J.A. and Platt, D. (eds) *The Child's World: The Essential Guide to Assessing Vulnerable Children, Young People and their Families* (3rd edition). London: Jessica Kingsley.

Bowyer, S. (2015) *Confident Practice with Cultural Diversity*. Totnes, Devon: Research in Practice.

Brackenridge, C. (2001) *Spoilsports: Understanding and Preventing Sexual Exploitation in Sport*. London: Routledge.

Brandon, M., Sidebotham, P., Belderson, P., Cleaver, H., Dickens, J., Garstan, J., Harris, J., Sorensen, P. and Wate, R. (2020) *Complexity and Challenge: A Triennial Analysis of SCRs 2014–2017*. London: Department for Education.

Broadley, K. (2019) 'Decision-making guidelines for the child protection intake phase'. In Bryce, I., Robinson, Y. and Petherick, W. (eds) *Child Abuse and Neglect: Forensic Issues in Evidence, Impact and Management*. London: Academic Press.

Bronfenbrenner, U. (1979) *The Ecology of Human Development: Experiments by Nature and Design*. Cambridge, MA: Harvard University Press.

Bronfenbrenner, U. (1991) 'What do families do?' *Institute for American Values*, Winter/Spring: 2.

Brown, J. (1999) 'Bowen family systems theory and practice: illustration and critique', *Australian and New Zealand Journal of Family Therapy*, 20(2): 94–103.

Butler-Sloss, E. (1988) *Report of the Inquiry into Child Abuse in Cleveland 1987*. London: HMSO.

Bywaters, P. (2013) 'Inequalities in child welfare: towards a new policy, research and action agenda', *British Journal of Social Work*, 45(1): 6–23.

Bywaters, P., Brady, G., Sparks, T. and Bos, E. (2016a) 'Child welfare inequalities: new evidence, further questions', *Child and Family Social Work*, 21: 369–80.

Bywaters, P., Bunting, L., Davidson, G., Hanratty, J., Mason, W., McCartan, C. and Steils, N. (2016b) *The Relationship between Poverty, Child Abuse and Neglect: An Evidence Review*. York: Joseph Rowntree Foundation.

Calderdale Safeguarding Children Partnership. Available at: https://safeguarding. calderdale.gov.uk/professionals/safeguarding-children/neglect/ (accessed 16 June 2020).

Canavan, J., Dolan, P. and Pinkerton, J. (2006) *Family Support: Direction from Diversity*. London: Jessica Kingsley.

Canavan, J., Pinkerton, J. and Dolan, P. (2016) *Understanding Family Support: Policy, Practice and Theory*. London: Jessica Kingsley.

Child Safeguarding Review Panel (2020) *It Was Hard to Escape: Safeguarding Children at Risk from Criminal Exploitation*. London: CSRP.

Cohen, S. (1972) *Folk Devils and Moral Panics*. London: Routledge.

Colver, A.F., Hutchinson, P.J. and Judson, E.C. (1982) 'Promoting children's home safety', *British Medical Journal*, 285(6349): 1177–80.

Corrigan, P. and Leonard, P. (1978) *Social Work Practice under Capitalism: A Marxist Approach*. London: Macmillan.

Crenshaw, K. (1990) 'Mapping the margins: intersectionality, identity politics, and violence against women of color', *Stanford Law Review*, *43*(6): 1241–99.

Cunningham, H. (2014) *Children and Childhood in Western Society since 1500*. London: Routledge.

Daly, M., Bruckhauf, Z., Byrne, J., Pecnik, N., Samms-Vaughan, M., Bray, R. and Margaria, A. (2015) *Family and Parenting Support: Policy and Provision in a Global Context*. Florence: UNICEF.

Davis, K. (2008) 'Intersectionality as buzzword: a sociology of science perspective on what makes a feminist theory successful', *Feminist Theory*, *9*(1): 67–85.

DeMause, L. (1974) *The History of Childhood*. New York: Psychohistory Press.

Department for Education (DfE) (2016) *Government Response to the Wood Review*. London: Department for Education.

Department for Education (DfE) (2017) *Child Sexual Exploitation: Definition and Guide for Practitioners*. London: Department for Education.

Department of Health (2000) *Safeguarding Children Involved in Prostitution: Supplementary Guidance to Working Together to Safeguard Children*. London: Department of Health.

Dolan, P. and Frost, N. (eds) (2017) *Routledge Handbook of Global Child Welfare*. London: Routledge.

Durrant, J.E. (1996) 'The Swedish ban on corporal punishment: its history and effects'. In Frehsee, D.W., Horn, W. and Bussman K.-D. (eds) *Family Violence against Children: A Challenge for Society*. New York: Walter de Gruyter.

Earle, F., Fox, J., Webb, C. and Bowyer, S. (2017) *Reflective Supervision: Resource Pack*. Totnes, Devon: Research in Practice.

Easton, C., Featherstone G., Poet, H., Aston, H., Gee, G. and Durbin, B. (2012) *Supporting Families with Complex Needs: Findings from LARC4*. Slough: NFER.

Ennew, J. (1986) *The Sexual Exploitation of Children*. Cambridge: Polity Press.

Eraut, M. (2012) 'Developing a broader approach to professional learning'. In McKee, A. and Eraut, M. (eds) *Learning Trajectories, Innovation and Identity for Professional Development*. Dordrecht: Springer.

Erooga, M. (2009) *Towards Safer Organisations: Adults Who Pose a Risk to Children in the Workplace and Implications for Recruitment and Selection*. London: NSPCC.

Featherstone, B., Gupta, A., Morris, K. and White, S. (2018) *Protecting Children: A Social Model*. Bristol: Policy Press.

Featherstone, B., White, S. and Morris, K. (2014) *Re-inventing Child Protection*. Bristol: Policy Press.

Feinstein, R.A. (2018) *When Rape was Legal: The Untold History of Sexual Violence During Slavery*. London: Routledge.

Felitti, V.J., Anda, R.F., Nordenberg, D., Williamson, D.F., Spitz, A.M., Edwards, V., Koss, M.P. and Marks, J.S. (1998) 'The relationship of adult health status to childhood abuse and household dysfunction', *American Journal of Preventive Medicine*, *14*: 245–58.

Ferguson, H. (2004) *Protecting Children in Time: Child Abuse, Child Protection and the Consequences of Modernity*. Basingstoke: Palgrave Macmillan.

Ferguson, H. (2011) *Child Protection Practice*. Basingstoke: Palgrave Macmillan.

Field-Fisher, T.G. (1974) *Report of the Committee of Inquiry into the Care and Supervision Provided in Relation to Maria Colwell*. London: HMSO.

Finkelhor, D. (1984) *Child Sexual Abuse: New Theory and Research*. New York: Sage.

Finkelhor, D. (2018) 'Screening for adverse childhood experiences (ACEs): cautions and suggestions', *Child Abuse & Neglect*, *85*: 174–9.

Finkelhor, D. and Browne, A. (1985) 'The traumatic impact of child sexual abuse: a conceptualization', *American Journal of Orthopsychiatry*, *55*(4): 530–41.

Firmin, C. (2017) *Abuse between Young People: A Contextual Account*. London: Routledge.

Fox, C. (2016) *'It's Not on the Radar': The Hidden Diversity of Children and Young People at Risk of Sexual Exploitation in England*. Barkingside: Barnardo's.

Fox-Harding, L. (2014) *Perspectives in Child Care Policy*. London: Routledge.

Freud, S. (1901) *The Psychopathology of Everyday Life*. New York: W.W. Norton & Company.

Frost, N. (2016) 'Learning from child protection Serious Case Reviews in England: a critical appraisal', *Social Work & Social Sciences Review*, *18*(3): 1–8.

Frost, N. (2019) 'Providing support and therapy for victims and survivors of child sexual exploitation', *Journal of Public Mental Health*, *18*(1): 38–45.

Frost, N., Abbott, S. and Race, T. (2015) *Family Support: Prevention, Early Intervention and Early Help*. Cambridge: Polity Press.

Frost, N. and Jackson, B. (2018) 'Research, policy and practice'. In Edwards, D. and Parkinson, K. (eds) *Family Group Conferences in Social Work: Involving Families in Social Care Decision Making*. Bristol: Policy Press.

Frost, N., Johnson, L., Stein, M. and Wallis, L. (2000) 'Home-start and the delivery of family support', *Children and Society*, *14*(5): 328–42.

Frost, N., Mills, S. and Stein, M. (1999) *Understanding Residential Child Care*. London: Ashgate Publishing Limited.

Frost, N. and Parton, N. (2009) *Understanding Children's Social Care: Politics, Policy and Practice*. London: Sage.

Frost, N. and Robinson, M. (2016) *Developing Multi-Professional Teamwork for Integrated Children's Services*. London: OUP.

Frost, N. and Stein, M. (1989) *The Politics of Child Welfare: Inequality, Power and Change*. Brighton: Harvester Wheatsheaf.

Fryer, P. (1997) '"Everybody's on Top of the Pops": popular music on British television 1960–1985', *Popular Music & Society, 21*(3): 153–71.

Gallagher, B. (2000) 'The extent and nature of known cases of institutional child sexual abuse', *British Journal of Social Work, 30*(6): 795–817.

Garrett, P.M. (2010) 'Examining the "conservative revolution": neoliberalism and social work education', *Social Work Education, 29*(4): 340–55.

Ghaffar, W., Manby, M. and Race, T. (2012) 'Exploring the experiences of parents and carers whose children have been subject to child protection plans', *British Journal of Social Work, 42*(5): 887–905.

Gibbs, G. (1988) *Learning by Doing: A Guide to Teaching and Learning Methods*. Oxford: Further Education Unit.

Gilligan, R. (2000) 'Adversity, resilience and young people: the protective value of positive school and spare time experiences', *Children and Society, 14*(1): 37–47.

Girl A (2013) *Girl A: My Story. The Truth about the Rochdale Sex Ring by the Victim Who Stopped Them*. London: Edbury Press.

Godar, R. (2013) *Commissioning Early Help*. Dartington: Research in Practice.

Goffman, E. (1961) *Asylums: Essays on the Social Situation of Mental Patients and other Inmates*. Harmondsworth: Penguin.

Gordon, L. (1988) *Heroes of Their Own Lives*. New York: Viking.

Gould, J. (2007) *Can't Buy Me Love: The Beatles, Britain and America*. London: Portrait.

Greer, C. and McLaughlin, E. (2013) 'The Sir Jimmy Savile scandal: child sexual abuse and institutional denial at the BBC', *Crime, Media, Culture, 9*(3): 243–63.

Hallett, S. (2017) *Making Sense of Child Sexual Exploitation: Exchange, Abuse and Young People*. Bristol: Policy Press.

Hanson, E. (2016) *Exploring the Relationship between Neglect and Child Sexual Exploitation*. Totnes, Devon: Research in Practice.

Hardiker, P., Exton, K. and Barker, M. (1991) *Policies and Practices in Preventive Child Care*. Aldershot: Gower.

Harlow, E. (2019) 'Attachment theory: developments, debates and recent applications in social work, social care and education', *Journal of Social Work Practice*. DOI: 10.1080/02650533.2019.1700493.

Hartill, M. (2014) 'Exploring narratives of boyhood sexual subjection in male-sport', *Sociology of Sport, 31*(1): 23–43.

Hill, P. (2016) 'Multi-agency working to safeguard children from sexual exploitation'. In: Frost, N. and Robinson, M. (eds) *Developing Multi-Professional Teamwork for Integrated Children's Services*. London: OUP

HMG (2015) *Working Together to Safeguard Children*. London: HMG.

HMG (2018) *Working Together to Safeguard Children*. London: HMG.

HMICFRSC (2020) *Both Sides of the Coin*. London: HMICFRSC.

Holmes, D. (2019) Transitional Safeguarding. Unpublished PowerPoint presentation.

Home Office (2018a) *Criminal Exploitation of Children and Vulnerable Adults: County Lines Guidance*. London: Home Office.

Home Office (2018b) *Serious Violence Strategy*. London: Home Office.

Horwath, J. (2007) *Child Neglect: Identification and Assessment*. Basingstoke: Macmillan International Higher Education.

Horwath, J. and Platt, D. (eds) (2019) *The Child's World: The Essential Guide to Assessing Vulnerable Children, Young People and their Families* (3rd edition). London: Jessica Kingsley.

Howard, K. and Brooks-Gunn, J. (2009) 'The role of home-visiting programs in preventing child abuse and neglect', *Future of Children, 19*(2): 119–46.

IICSA (2018) *Ampleforth and Downside Report*. London: Independent Inquiry into Child Sexual Abuse.

ILO (1999) *Worst Forms of Child Labour Convention*. Geneva: ILO.

INSPIRE/WHO (2018) *INSPIRE: Seven strategies for Ending Violence Against Children*. Available at: https://www.who.int/publications/i/item/inspire-seven-strategies-for-ending-violence-against-children (accessed 16 June 2020).

Jago, S., Arocha, L., Brodie, I., Melrose, M., Pearce, J.J. and Warrington, C. (2011) *What's Going on to Safeguard Children and Young People from Sexual Exploitation? How Local Partnerships Respond to Child Sexual Exploitation*. Luton: University of Bedfordshire.

Jay, A. (2014) *Independent Inquiry into Child Sexual Exploitation in Rotherham: 1997–2013*. Rotherham: Rotherham Metropolitan Borough Council.

Johnson, R., Browne, K. and Hamilton-Giachritsis, C. (2006) 'Young children in institutional care at risk of harm', *Trauma, Violence and Abuse, 7*(1): 34–60.

Jones, R. (2014) *The Story of Baby P: Setting the Record Straight*. Bristol: Policy Press.

Kelly, L. and Karsna, K. (2017) 'Measuring the scale and changing nature of child sexual abuse and child sexual exploitation. Scoping report'. Barkingside: Centre of Expertise on Child Sexual Abuse.

Kempe, C.H. (1971) 'Paediatric implications of the battered baby syndrome', *Archives of Disease in Childhood, 46*(245): 28–37.

Kempe, C.H., Silverman, F.N., Steele, B.F., Droegemueller, W. and Silver, H.K. (2013) 'The battered-child syndrome'. In Krugman, R.D. and Korbin, J.E. (eds) *C. Henry Kempe: A 50 Year Legacy to the Field of Child Abuse and Neglect*. Dordrecht: Springer.

Kirby, P. (2003) *Child Labour in Britain, 1750–1870*. Basingstoke: Macmillan International Higher Education.

Knight, C. (2019) 'Trauma informed practice and care: implications for field instruction', *Clinical Social Work Journal, 47*(1): 79–89.

Krugman, R.D. and Korbin, J.E. (eds) (2012) *C. Henry Kempe: A 50 Year Legacy to the Field of Child Abuse and Neglect*. Dordrecht: Springer.

Laming (2003) *The Victoria Climbié Inquiry: Report of an Inquiry by Lord Laming*. Norwich: TSO.

Lefevre, M., Hickle, K. and Luckock, B. (2019) '"Both/and" not "either/or": reconciling rights to protection and participation in working with child sexual Exploitation', *British Journal of Social Work, 49*(7): 1837–54.

Leigh, J. and Laing, J. (2018) *Thinking about Child Protection Practice: Case Studies for Critical Reflection and Discussion*. Bristol: Policy Press.

Local Government Association (2017) *Tackling Modern Slavery: A Council Guide*. London: LGA

Lovett, J., Coy, M. and Kelly, L. (2018) *Deflection, Denial and Disbelief: Social and Political Discourses about Child Sexual Abuse and their Influence on Institutional Responses. A Rapid Evidence Assessment*. London: IICSA.

Lynch, M.A. (1985) 'Child abuse before Kempe: an historical literature review', *Child Abuse & Neglect, 9*(1): 7–15.

Marre, D. and Briggs, L. (eds) (2009) *International Adoption: Global Inequalities and the Circulation of Children*. New York: New York University Press.

Marx, K. (1852) *The Eighteenth Brumaire of Louis Bonaparte*. London: Wildside Press.

McNeish, D. and Scott, S. (2018) *Key Messages from Research into Institutional Child Sexual Abuse*. Barkingside: Centre of Expertise on Child Sexual Abuse.

Meissner, F. and Vertovec, S. (2015) 'Comparing super-diversity', *Ethnic and Racial Studies, 38*(4): 541–55.

Middleton, J. (2008) 'The experience of corporal punishment in schools, 1890–1940', *History of Education, 37*(2): 253–75.

Miller, D. and Brown, J. (2014) *'We Have the Right to Be Safe': Protecting Disabled Children from Abuse*. London: NSPCC.

Ministry of Justice (2011) *Achieving Best Evidence in Criminal Proceedings*. London: Ministry of Justice.

Morrison, T. (1993) *Staff Supervision in Social Care: An Action Learning Approach*. London: Longman.

Munro, E. (1999) 'Protecting children in an anxious society', *Health, Risk & Society, 1*(1), 117–27.

Munro, E. (2005) 'A systems approach to investigating child abuse deaths', *British Journal of Social Work, 35*(4): 531–46.

Munro, E. (2011) *The Munro Review of Child Protection: Final Report, A Child-Centred System* (Vol. *8062*). London: The Stationery Office.

Nelson, S. (2016) *Tackling Child Sexual Abuse: Radical Approaches to Prevention, Protection and Support*. Bristol: Policy Press.

NICE (n.d.) *The Health Needs of Unaccompanied Asylum Seeking Children and Young People*, prepared by Simmonds, J. and Meredew, F. London: NICE.

Nicholas, J. (2015) *Practical Guide to Child Protection*. London: Jessica Kingsley.

North Yorkshire County Council (2014) *Domestic Abuse Youth Support Services Guidelines*. Northallerton: North Yorkshire County Council.

NSPCC (2013) *Domestic Abuse*. London: NSPCC.

NSPCC (2018) *How Safe Are Our Children?* London: NSPCC.

OCC (2011) 'Thousands of sexually exploited children in England: OCC Inquiry launched into Child Sexual Exploitation in Gangs and Groups (CSEGG)'. Press Release, 14 October, Office of the Children's Commissioner for England.

OCC (2019) 'Keeping kids safe: improving safeguarding responses to gang violence and criminal exploitation', February. London: Office of the Children's Commissioner for England. Available at: www.childrenscommissioner.gov.uk/report/keeping-kids-safe/ (accessed 5 August 2020).

Ofsted (2016) *Time to Listen: A Joined Up Response to Child Sexual Exploitation and Missing Children*. London: Ofsted.

Pace (2019) *The Relational Safeguarding Model: Best Practice in Working with Families Affected by Child Exploitation* (3rd edition). Leeds: Pace.

Parton, N. (1985) *The Politics of Child Abuse*. Basingstoke: Macmillan.

Parton, N. (2010) 'From dangerousness to risk: the growing importance of screening and surveillance systems for safeguarding and promoting the well-being of children in England', *Health, Risk & Society*, 12(1): 51–64.

Parton, N. (2017) 'Comparing child protection systems'. In Dolan, P. and Frost, N. (eds) *Routledge Handbook of Global Child Welfare*. London: Routledge.

Pearson, G. (1983) *Hooligan: A History of Respectable Fears*. Basingstoke: Macmillan International Higher Education.

Pike, C. (2019) *Prey: My Fight to Survive the Halifax Grooming Gang*. London: John Blake Publishing.

Pinkerton, J. and Katz, I. (2003) 'Perspective through international comparison in the evaluation of family support'. In Katz, I. and Pinkerton, J. (eds) *Evaluating Family Support: Thinking Internationally, Thinking Critically*. London: Wiley.

Pollock, L.A. (1983) *Forgotten Children: Parent–Child Relations from 1500 to 1900*. Cambridge: Cambridge University Press.

Pritchard, C. and Williams, R. (2009) 'Comparing possible "child-abuse-related-deaths" in England and Wales with the major developed countries 1974–2006: signs of progress?', *British Journal of Social Work*, 40(6): 1700–22.

Public Health England (2019) *Child Sexual Exploitation: How Public Health Can Support Prevention and Intervention*. London: Public Health England.

Pugh, G. (2011) *London's Forgotten Children: Thomas Coram and the Foundling Hospital*. London: The History Press.

Race, T. (2019) 'Hearing the voice of the child in child protection processes'. PhD thesis, Leeds Beckett University.

Race, T. and O'Keefe, R. (2017) *Child-Centred Practice: A Handbook for Social Work*. London: Macmillan International Higher Education.

Raj, A. and McDougal, L. (2014) 'Sexual violence and rape in India', *Lancet*, *383*(9920): 865.

Re D (A Child) (No. 3) [2016] EWFC 1.

Rees, G. and Stein, M. (1999) *The Abuse of Adolescents within the Family*. London: NSPCC. http://eprints.whiterose.ac.uk/75149/1/Document.pdf.

Rikala, S. (2019) 'Agency among young people in marginalised positions: towards a better understanding of mental health problems', *Journal of Youth Studies, 2019*: 1–17.

Robinson, W.S. (2012) *Muckraker: The Scandalous Life and Times of W. T. Stead, Britain's First Investigative Journalist*. London: Biteback Publishing.

Saunders, H. (2004) *Twenty-Nine Child Homicides*. Bristol: Women's Aid Federation of England.

Schweinhart, L., Montie, J., Xiang, Z., Barnett, W., Bellfield, C. and Nores, M. (2005) *Lifetime Effects: The HighScope Perry Pre-School Study through age 40*. Ypsilanti, MI: HighScope Press.

Seabrook, D. (2006) *White Heat*. London: Little, Brown.

Shaheed, F. (2012) *Engaging Resistant, Challenging and Complex Families*. Totnes, Devon: Research in Practice.

Shannon, M. (2019) *Family Support for Social Care Practitioners*. London: Red Globe Press.

Sharland, E. (2006) 'Young people, risk taking and risk making: some thoughts for social work', *British Journal of Social Work*, 36(2): 247–65.

Shaw, P. (2016) *Communicating with Children and Young People with Speech, Language and Communication Needs and/or Developmental Delay*. Totnes, Devon: Research in Practice.

Skinner, B.F. (1971) *Beyond Freedom and Dignity*. New York: Knopf.

Smith, Dame Janet (2016a) *The Jimmy Savile Investigation Report, Volume Two*. London: BBC.

Smith, Dame Janet (2016b) *The Stuart Hall Investigation Report, Volume Three*. London: BBC.

Snow, R.P. (1987) 'Youth, rock'n'roll, and electronic media', *Youth and Society*, 18(4), 326–43.

Spicer, J., Moyle, L. and Coomber, R. (2019) 'The variable and evolving nature of "cuckooing" as a form of criminal exploitation in street level drug markets', *Trends in Organized Crime, 2019*: 1–23. https://link.springer.com/article/10.1007/s12117-019-09368-5.

Stead, W.T. (1885) 'The Maiden Tribute of Modern Babylon I: The Report of our Secret Commission', *Pall Mall Gazette*.

Stedman Jones, G. (2014) *Outcast London: A Study in the Relationship between Classes in Victorian Society*. London: Verso.

Stewart, J. (1995) 'Children, parents and the state: the Children Act, 1908', *Children & Society, 9*(1): 90–9.

Taylor, D. (2017) 'One year after football's child abuse scandal broke, stories are yet to be told', *The Observer*, 11 November. Available at: www.theguardian.com/football/2017/nov/11/andy-woodward-one-year-on (accessed 26 July 2018).

Taylor-Robinson, D.C., Straatmann, V.S. and Whitehead, M. (2018) 'Adverse childhood experiences or adverse childhood socioeconomic conditions?', *The Lancet Public Health, 3*(6): 262–3.

Ungaretti, J.R. (1978) 'Pederasty, heroism, and the family in classical Greece', *Journal of Homosexuality, 3*(3): 291–300.

Warren, W.A. (2007) '"The cause of her grief": the rape of a slave in Early New England', *The Journal of American History, 93*(4): 1031–49.

Watkins, S.A. (1990) 'The Mary Ellen myth: correcting child welfare history', *Social Work, 35*(6): 500–3.

Weale, S. (2020) 'Youth services suffer 70% funding cut in less than a decade', *The Guardian*, 20 January.

Wenger, E. (1999) *Communities of Practice: Learning, Meaning, and Identity*. Cambridge: Cambridge University Press.

Whitzman, C. (2016) '"Culture eats strategy for breakfast": the powers and limitations of urban design education', *Journal of Urban Design, 21*(5): 574–6.

Wilkinson, R. and Pickett, K. (2009) *The Spirit Level: Why Equality is Better for Everyone*. London: Penguin.

Wood, A. (2016) *Review of the Role and Functions of LSCBs*. London: Department for Education.

Woolcock, G. (2016) 'The development and production of local, national and international state of children's well-being report cards'. In Kee, Y., Lee, S.J. and Phillips, R. (eds) *Social Factors and Community Well-Being*. Cham: Springer.

Wright, H.R. (2015) *The Child in Society*. London: Sage.

INDEX